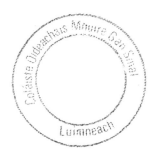

Cognitive Analysis
of Dyslexia

International Library of Psychology

Cognitive Analysis of Dyslexia

Philip H.K. Seymour

Routledge & Kegan Paul

London and New York

First published in 1986
by Routledge & Kegan Paul plc

11 New Fetter Lane, London EC4P 4EE,

Published in the USA by
Routledge & Kegan Paul Inc.
in association with Methuen Inc.
29 West 35th Street, New York, NY 10001

Set in Baskerville 10/12pt
by Columns, Reading
and printed by
St Edmundsbury Press, Bury St Edmunds, Suffolk

Library of Congress Cataloging in Publication Data
Seymour, Philip H. K. (Philip Herschel Kean), 1938–

Cognitive analysis of dyslexia.
(International library of psychology)
Bibliography: p.
Includes index.
1. Dyslexia. 2. Cognition. I. Title. II. Series.
RJ496.A5S49 1986   616.85'53   86-419

British Library CIP data also available

ISBN 0-7100-9841-3

for Jane

Contents

Preface

I have for some years been interested in the idea that reading difficulties might beneficially be analysed by an application of the theories and methods of experimental cognitive psychology. This monograph provides an account of part of a project, carried out with support from the Medical Research Council, in which I explored the scope of such an application. The book is not a general treatise on the topic of dyslexia. Nor is it a comprehensive discussion of the cognitive psychology of reading. I have instead restricted myself to a presentation of the data obtained in the course of an experimental investigation of the reading processes of competent and developmentally dyslexic individuals, and the explication of a particular scheme of cognitive interpretation. The research has not revealed the fundamental causes of dyslexia. It has, on the other hand, been helpful in delineating the consequences of the disorder for the development of a partially operational reading system in individual cases. It is my hope that this kind of clarification can contribute to the diagnosis and, ultimately, the remediation of reading difficulties.

Dundee
June 1985

Acknowledgments

The research described in this volume was carried out with the support of a grant from the Medical Research Council of the UK. The work benefited greatly from the co-operation of the Tayside Dyslexia Association.

I am most grateful to the subjects for their tolerance in submitting themselves to a lengthy series of experimental studies; to Jane MacGregor and Penny Balfour for their assistance with the testing; to Carol Ervine for the psycho-educational assessments; and to Anna Spackman for help with the preparation of the manuscript. Thanks are also due to Patrick Seymour for writing the clock routine for the Apple II computer, and to Penny Balfour for drawing the figures.

1 A cognitive approach

1.1 Definition of 'dyslexia'

'Dyslexia', defined as a disability affecting the uses of written language, has been acknowledged since the publication of various pioneering investigations during the nineteenth century. The classical studies of Déjerine established that dyslexia could occur in adulthood as a consequence of damage to particular areas of the brain and that an acquired reading disorder of this type might or might not be accompanied by a dysgraphia (a disorder of writing and spelling) (Geschwind, 1965). Other authors, particularly Hinshelwood (1917), presented case studies illustrating that reading difficulties might also occur congenitally, that is as an impairment of the development during childhood of basic reading and orthographic skills in the absence of evidence of neurological trauma as a precipitating factor.

There is, therefore, a need to distinguish between 'acquired dyslexia' resulting from damage incurred by the brain following the earlier establishment of normal reading and spelling competence, and 'developmental dyslexia', referring to a disruption of reading and spelling acquisition during childhood. This monograph will be concerned almost exclusively with the analysis of developmental dyslexia although evidence and concepts deriving from studies of acquired dyslexia will be considered when relevant.

The definition of 'dyslexia' has been the subject of an acrimonious and arguably futile debate. This stems from a wish on the part of some people to use the term to refer exclusively to children whose reading or spelling disorder is highly specific and surprising in the context of their circumstances and other abilities. Others take the contrary view that this special group cannot reliably be distinguished from the general run of children who have difficulty in learning to read and spell. The problem is well illustrated by a consideration of the oft-quoted definition proposed by the members of a congress of neurologists at a meeting held in 1968.

1

Critchley (1970) summarised this definition in the following terms:

> *Specific developmental dyslexia* A disorder manifested by difficulty in learning to read despite conventional instruction, adequate intelligence, and socio-cultural opportunity. It is dependent upon fundamental cognitive disabilities which are frequently of constitutional origin.

It can be seen that there are two parts to this statement. The first is a definition by exclusion which advises neurologists that a diagnosis of dyslexia might most confidently be made when a severe reading disability was found to occur in the absence of other negative influences, such as poor general intelligence, poor socio-economic standing, or disrupted or inadequate schooling. The second part asserts that the disorder is dependent on fundamental 'cognitive disabilities' which may well have their origin in the genetic programming of the development of the brain in early life. Since genetic influences of this kind cannot be expected to respect the boundaries of poor intelligence, poor social circumstances or poor schooling, it is implicit that dyslexic problems may occur at any level of intelligence, social status or adequacy of schooling. It follows that the definition by exclusion contained in the first part of the statement is no more than an admission that 'dyslexia' is easier to diagnose in children who are intellectually, socially and educationally advantaged than in those who are not.

On these grounds I would argue that the restrictive use of the term 'dyslexia' constitutes a category mistake. It involves a pragmatically motivated stipulation that a general term should be applied restrictively to a subset of the larger class to which it refers. My own view is that no useful purpose is served by promulgating or seeking to defend this stipulation or indeed by arguing about its validity. In this monograph the term 'dyslexia' will be used simply as a label for a disturbance affecting the establishment of basic reading and spelling skills. Dyslexia is defined as 'difficulty in learning to read'.

I will take 'learning to read' to mean the setting up of a basic competence in both reading and spelling, where 'basic competence' refers to those behavioural demonstrations which are generally acceptable as an indication that an individual has established the fundamentals of reading and spelling – for example, the ability to read out and show comprehension of familiar visual words, or the ability to reproduce the conventional spelling of a word on demand.

It has been the contribution of educational psychologists such as Burt and Schonell to compile graded word lists which can be used to assess this basic level of competence and to provide age-related norms which define a public standard of adequacy. If the tests and their norms can be accepted as a legitimate metric of competence, then the term 'dyslexia' might be considered to be applicable whenever a child's performance was shown to deviate by some criterial amount below the norm for his age.

1.2 Cognitive level of analysis

The second part of Critchley's (1970) definition asserts that 'dyslexia' is dependent on 'fundamental cognitive disabilities'. I would suggest that this element of the definition points to a psychological level of analysis and that this level should be distinguished from the level of competence considered in the preceding section. At the level of competence it is sufficient to assert that an individual cannot demonstrate the behaviours which are considered to underpin the public concept of literacy and that the designation 'dyslexic' is accordingly appropriate. If a second, psychological level of description is invoked, this carries with it the implied assumption that the behaviours from which reading and spelling competence are inferred are the products of a set of underlying psychological processes, and that, in cases of dyslexia, certain of these processes operate in an atypical or defective manner. This second level of description can in its turn be reformulated at a third physiological level. The assumption here is that psychological processes are, ultimately, brain processes which are instantiated within the medium of the central nervous system and its associated receptor and effector organs.

These three possible levels of description and explanation can be summarised in the following terms:

Level I Competence
A statement of the publicly observable behaviours which define the concept of 'literacy' (ability to read and spell) and of the failures to demonstrate these behaviours at a criterial level of adequacy which define the concept of 'dyslexia'.

Level II Cognitive function
An analysis, stated in functional (information processing) terms of psychological processes underlying the behaviours which define 'literacy' and of the manner in which these are modified or distorted in cases of 'dyslexia'.

Level III Physiological instantiation
An account of the manner in which the mental functions underlying competence are realised in neural tissue and localised in brain structure and of physiological distinctions (including receptor and effector activities) existing between dyslexic and normally competent individuals.

Arguments can be put forward to justify investigations of dyslexia at each of these three levels. To some extent the choice of level has been conditioned by the specialism from which a researcher approaches the topic. Educational psychology has typically been concerned with the assessment of competence, generally by the application of standardised test instruments, and has focused on the analysis of dyslexia at Level I, especially questions about the relationship between literacy and other aspects of human intelligence. Medically related disciplines, like neuropsychology, are naturally concerned with the investigation of questions formulated at Level III, such as whether dyslexic children are characterised by atypical brain development, the possibility of a relationship between dyslexia and cerebral dominance, or the role of atypical auditory, visual or oculomotor processes in dyslexia.

The research to be described in this monograph differs from most previously reported investigations in being formulated with the explicit and almost exclusive intention of carrying out an analysis at Level II, the level of description of cognitive processes. Such an approach may ultimately be shown to be vulnerable to objections of a fundamental philosophical character regarding the status of Level II descriptions in a theory of mind. For the present, however, there exists a branch of cognitive science, which I will refer to as 'experimental cognitive psychology', which has as its objective the development of empirical procedures capable of providing the data necessary to underpin theories which are formulated at the second level of description. My own ideas regarding this enterprise have been set out in an earlier publication (Seymour, 1979). By a Level II (cognitive) approach I refer to attempts to apply the theories and methods of experimental cognitive psychology to the investigation of the reading processes of dyslexic subjects.

1.3 A two-channel model

My concern with 'dyslexia' dates from a period in the mid-1970s. At about that time a voluntary organisation, the Tayside Dyslexia Association, was formed in Dundee by parents and teachers with interests, often of a direct and personal nature, in the provision of help for children with severe reading and spelling difficulties. A PhD student working under my supervision coincidentally decided to switch to dyslexia as the topic of his research.

My own interests were at that time directed towards the theoretical and experimental analysis of normal cognitive functions (Seymour, 1979). I had been particularly concerned with questions about the manner in which pictorial, spatial and temporal concepts might be represented in semantic memory and the nature of the process of accessing this type of information from verbal or pictorial input. The 'logogen model' formulated by John Morton provided a convenient framework for identification of cognitive systems which might be involved in the performance of tasks such as reading, comprehension, object naming and verification (Morton, 1968; Seymour, 1973). My inclination, when confronted with my student's questions about the basis of dyslexic difficulties, was to consider whether the problem could be represented within the information processing framework exemplified by the logogen model, and whether properties of dyslexic reading could be analysed using currently available cognitive experimental methods.

The study carried out by my student involved an information processing analysis of the reading functions of four dyslexic boys and two dyslexic adults. From the account published by Seymour and Porpodas (1980) it can be seen that a 'two-channel model' of both reading and spelling was employed as a framework to guide the selection of experimental tasks and the interpretation of results. This theory asserts that the interpretation of an array of letters typically involves the co-operation of two functionally distinct processes: a lexical process, by which the pronunciation of known words may be directly 'looked up' or addressed, and a non-lexical process which makes use of a knowledge of letter-sound associations to assemble a conventionally acceptable pronunciation.

The two-channel theory is fundamental to the psycholinguistic analysis of basic reading processes which is currently popular in cognitive psychology and neuropsychology. The assumption is made that the various functional components contained within an information processing system may be sensitive to differing properties of language. These properties, which include the frequencies of occurrence of words, the concrete or abstract nature of their meaning, and the regularity of their pronunciation, can be varied by a judicious selection of materials. According to the two-channel theory, the lexical process is capable of recognising familiar words but not letter arrays, which, although conventionally spelled, are not known words. The non-lexical process is considered to be capable of translating words which contain standard spelling-to-sound correspondences but not those which contain atypical or irregular spellings (Coltheart, 1978). It follows from these assumptions that two factors which are particularly important in a psycholinguistic analysis of reading functions are: (1) lexicality, the distinction between known words and non-words, and (2) spelling-to-sound regularity, an index of the degree to which the letters contained in a word receive a conventional pronunciation.

In the Seymour and Porpodas study a psycholinguistic analysis of reading functions was combined with an information processing analysis. By this I mean an application of the method which is standard in experimental cognitive psychology, involving tests of the effects on speed and accuracy of response of systematic variations in factors considered relevant to the operation of the information processing system. For example, a consideration of the effects on reading reaction time of variations in word length may be informative in relation to questions about the serial or parallel nature of the process which handles the letters making up a word during recognition.

1.4 Presumption in favour of heterogeneity

At the time when Costas Porpodas was conducting his research, it was not clear to me whether developmental dyslexia should be regarded as a unitary condition, perhaps varying in severity, or whether it was reasonable to anticipate that distinctive patterns might exist. A prevailing assumption in cognitive psychology seemed to be that normal adult reading could plausibly be regarded as a unitary phenomenon. This presumption justified research in which reading processes were investigated by conducting series of discrete experiments on subject groups of changing personnel and by drawing conclusions from statistical analyses of group data in which individual differences were treated as error variance.

It has been quite common for investigators of reading acquisition and disability to adopt a similar methodology. Questions about the course of normal development are addressed by making comparisons between groups of children of differing ages or competence. The nature of reading disability (dyslexia) is investigated by comparing results from groups of impaired readers with results from groups of normal readers of similar age or competence. Implicit in the adoption of this group methodology is the assumption that normal reading is a unitary phenomenon at each of its developmental levels and that the same is true of impaired reading.

I will refer to this theoretical standpoint and its associated methodology as the 'presumption in favour of homogeneity'. It is a presumption which is widely and almost unquestioningly held in cognitive psychology and one which directs what appears to be a natural and orthodox approach to the investigation of such topics as dyslexia. Nonetheless, it stands in fundamental contrast to the methodology which has been established in cognitive neuropsychology as a procedure for studying acquired disorders of reading and writing (and other cognitive functions).

In a pioneering paper, Marshall and Newcombe (1973) provided outline descriptions of six patients whose reading functions had been impaired following brain damage incurred during adulthood. An analysis of the errors they made and of the effects on their reading of psycholinguistic variables was used to support the proposal that a visual, phonological or semantic component of an information processing system underlying reading competence might be selectively impaired as a consequence of neurological damage, and that the pattern of disturbed performance observed could be expected to differ in theoretically coherent ways depending on which component was affected. A single case methodology was employed, with data from a small number of selected patients being used to illustrate the various theoretical possibilities.

At the time developmental dyslexia had not been analysed in quite the same way, although it was usual for some commentators, especially those working in the field of learning disabilities, to propose alternative types of disorder, sometimes referred to as 'visual dyslexia' and 'auditory dyslexia' (Johnson and Myklebust, 1967). Boder (1973) published an influential paper in which she argued on the basis of an analysis of the reading and spelling errors of individual children for the existence of two contrasting types, which she called 'dyseidetic dyslexia' and 'dysphonetic dyslexia'. At a fairly general qualitative level this appeared to correspond to the contrast between 'surface dyslexia' and 'deep dyslexia' which Marshall and Newcombe (1973) proposed in their analysis of cases of acquired dyslexia.

According to Marshall and Newcombe, 'surface dyslexia' is a condition in which there is a defect of word recognition and semantic access (the lexical process) combined with a relative preservation of the assembly of pronunciation by the application of letter-sound associations (the non-lexical process). 'Dyseidetic dyslexia' is a corresponding disturbance of the development of a word recognition system which results in an over-reliance on the use of grapheme-phoneme correspondences in both reading and spelling.

In 'deep dyslexia' there is an impairment of letter-sound associations although word recognition processes may be preserved, resulting in reading which is dependent on semantic mediation and which is characterised by semantic errors (for example, reading 'thunder' as 'storm') and by effects of variables such as concrete versus abstract meaning. 'Dysphonetic dyslexia' is a developmental disorder which affects the establishment of grapheme-phoneme correspondences. In practice, it may be more appropriate to think in terms of an analogy between this condition and acquired 'phonological dyslexia' (Beauvois and Derouesné, 1979), a disorder in which the use of grapheme-phoneme correspondences is impaired although the semantic anomalies characteristic of deep dyslexia (especially the semantic errors) do not occur.

If the possibility of theoretically significant differences among developmentally dyslexic children is a real one, then it follows that the orthodox methodology which attempts to establish general contrasts between groups of normal readers and groups of impaired readers may be of limited utility. What is required is an alternative methodology which is based on a 'presumption in favour of heterogeneity'. This is the presumption, adopted at the outset of research, that dyslexic subjects may possess individual processing characteristics, and that the identification and description of these characteristics represents a principal objective of investigation.

1.5 Dyslexic sub-types

In the study of the acquired dyslexias, the approach has been to identify individual patients who appear 'interesting' in the sense that they exhibit symptoms which are in some way surprising or clearly relevant to a current theoretical concern and then to undertake a detailed case study, possibly adapting the method 'on line' in response to particular observations. I will refer to this single case approach as the 'neuropsychological method'.

Researchers using this method appear to be committed both to the idea of single case studies and to the view that the dyslexic population, although heterogeneous, is capable of sub-division into a number of categories or sub-types. It is argued that a single case which displays interesting and theoretically coherent features can stand as a prototypical exemplar of a sub-type, much as Marshall and Newcombe's patient, GR, stands as a prototypical example of the category of deep dyslexia. As other cases are individually examined and reported, they may be found to yield similar data and hence to merit the same sub-type classification or to produce data which are, to a sufficient degree, different, and which are consequently capable of forcing the postulation of new sub-types (Coltheart, 1980).

The juxtaposition of this confidence in the existence of sub-types and commitment to a single case methodology is on the face of it surprising. A more usual way of attempting to establish the existence and identity of sub-types is to apply a battery of tests to a large sample of subjects and to use statistical procedures, such as factor analysis, in order to determine whether coherent groupings or dimensions of variation can be identified. This methodology has been widely used in educational research, often with the objective of isolating different types of learning disability (Satz and Morris, 1981) or reading disability (Mitterer, 1982).

It may be instructive to consider why neuropsychologists interested in the classification of acquired reading disorders did not follow this standard approach. Possibly the critical point is that the factor analytic procedure shares with the orthodox experimental methodology the property of being descriptive of groups and populations and not of the processing systems established in individual subjects. In cognitive neuropsychology the construction of individual processing descriptions is the primary objective whereas the possibility of grouping descriptions into sub-types is a secondary issue which is in any case subordinate to the requirements of theoretical coherence. An important additional point is that sub-type proposals in neuropsychology are dependent on the availability of Level II (cognitive) descriptions. They are, in this sense, semantic categories imposed on interpretations of data and not mathematical groupings waiting to be discovered within the raw data themselves.

I would argue, therefore, that a viable approach to the objective of determining whether or not sub-types of developmental dyslexia exist may be to construct cognitive descriptions of individual cases and then to proceed to consider to what extent the descriptions may be said to be the same as or different from one another. It should then be possible to adjudicate between the following outcomes:

Homogeneity
If developmental dyslexia is homogeneous all dyslexic cases will receive the same cognitive description.

Sub-types
If sub-types exist, there will be a small number of distinctively different descriptions, each shared by a number of individuals.

Heterogeneity
If the dyslexic population is heterogeneous each subject will receive a different cognitive description.

A choice among these three possible accounts of developmental dyslexia might be approached by adopting without modification the procedures which have been followed in the analysis of acquired dyslexia. This would involve the detailed study of developmental cases which revealed interesting features. Some researchers have taken the view that developmental cases may be deemed to be 'interesting' if they can be shown to share features with some of the acquired sub-types which have been identified. For example, Temple and Marshall (1983) reported details of a single case of developmental phonological dyslexia, and Coltheart, Byng, Masterson, Prior and Riddoch (1983) described the results of a subject whom they considered to be a case of developmental surface dyslexia.

My own view is that this approach is probably too selective and too esoteric to recommend itself as a general procedure for investigating reading disability in children. There is in the first place the danger that the categories of disorder which have been formulated in the description of acquired dyslexia will dominate the selection of cases and the interpretation of data. Secondly, the objective of research is presumably not simply the advancement of theoretical knowledge but also the development of an analysis of the broad run of reading disorders which are likely to be encountered in the classroom or educational clinic. It seems obvious that this more general objective cannot be served by restricting investigation to a small number of special cases which are characterised by intriguing features or purity of deficit or similarity to a category of acquired disorder.

On these grounds, I would argue that a sensible procedure to adopt in the analysis of developmental dyslexia is one which combines the cognitive investigation of individuals with an open-ended and non-selective approach to subject sampling.

1.6 Conclusions

In this preliminary chapter I have outlined the case for undertaking a cognitive analysis of developmental dyslexia. This task can be approached by following a series of steps, involving: (1) the formulation of a functional model of basic reading processes, (2) the setting up of an experimental procedure designed to investigate the component systems of the model, and (3) the application of the procedure to the individual members of samples of competent and dyslexic readers. The data should be open to interpretation within the terms of the model, leading to the production of Level II (cognitive) descriptions of each individual case. Once a sufficiently large number of such descriptions has been collected, it should become possible to comment on the degree of homogeneity or heterogeneity present in the dyslexic sample, and on the possibility that distinctive sub-types exist.

2 Information processing framework

2.1 Introduction

I applied in 1980 to the Medical Research Council of the UK for funds to support a two-year study of the 'Cognitive basis of spelling disability'. The *raison d'être* of this project was the observation, made by Critchley (1970), Miles (1983) and others, that dyslexic children often give evidence of cognitive disturbances other than difficulties with reading and spelling. These particularly affect the conceptualisation of space and time and are apparent as confusions between right and left, poor understanding of compass point direction, difficulty in learning to read the clock, poor mastery of the time labelling sequences (the days of the week or the months of the year) and problems in learning other conventional sequences such as the alphabet or the arithmetical tables. At the time that I made the proposal to the Medical Research Council it seemed to me possible that these areas of spatial and temporal knowledge might share with the storage of spelling a dependence on certain fundamental structures required for the coding of position, adjacency and direction within ordered arrays of elements, and that dyslexic problems stemmed from a disturbance of this representational system.

The Medical Research Council agreed to support a two-year project to study this problem. When the project began in the summer of 1981 I made the decision that the research should focus on older developmentally dyslexic subjects and that the analysis of spatial and temporal functions should be supported by a cognitive analysis of reading processes and spelling processes. This meant that there were three parts to the project, involving:

1   Analysis of basic reading processes, using cognitive experimental methods.
2   Analysis of spelling and writing functions, based on a consideration of spelling errors and the timing of writing movements.

11

3   A cognitive analysis of spatial and temporal representation, focusing particularly on clock time, the months and days series and simple arithmetical processes.

I propose in this monograph to restrict myself to a discussion of the first of these components, the analysis of basic reading functions. Once the description of reading processes is established, it will become possible to treat spelling and writing in the light of what is known about reading, and then to consider the spatial and temporal representational functions in the light of what is known about both.

This chapter and the next will describe the steps which were followed through in setting up a procedure for the cognitive analysis of reading functions. As was noted in Chapter 1, the first requirement is for a broadly defined functional model which can be used as an interpretative framework for research. The properties of such a model and the way in which it may be related to questions about reading development and disability will be explored in this chapter. The next step, which will be taken in Chapter 3, is to define a set of tasks and factor variations which are likely to be helpful in assessing the functioning of the model.

2.2 Functional analysis of basic reading processes

In Chapter 1, I argued that areas of human achievement, such as reading and spelling, could be analysed at three different levels, termed the level of competence, the level of cognitive function, and the level of physiological instantiation. In this monograph I shall not be concerned at all with the third (physiological) level of description. Some consideration of the first (competence) level is essential in order to determine the degree to which subjects fall within a public definition of 'dyslexia'. For this purpose I have relied in the main on reports prepared by educational psychologists and other professionals with interests in the assessment of reading disorders.

The first step in the construction of a Level II (cognitive) description is the formulation of an information processing model in which functionally defined systems are represented together with channels of communication between them. A prototypical example of such a scheme is provided by the 'logogen model' formulated by Morton (1968, 1969). This model, which was designed to offer an account of contextual influences on reading and listening, incorporated a suggestion that contact between incoming sensory information and centrally stored representations of meaning and speech might be mediated by a word (or morpheme)-specific recognition and retrieval system, which Morton called a 'logogen system'. Since that time many variants of this basic idea have been proposed. Most of these have had the effect of differentiating and elaborating the original scheme, by making explicit distinctions between recognition of input and production of output, between speech production and spelling production on the output side, or between spoken words, written words and pictures of objects on the input side. In addition, Morton and Patterson (1980) proposed that visually based access to speech might involve co-operation between a 'lexical process' and a non-lexical grapheme-phoneme translation process (i.e. the two-channel model utilised in the Seymour and Porpodas experiments).

Although I have contributed to the various debates about the structure of the logogen model (Seymour, 1973, 1979; Seymour and Porpodas, 1980), I do not wish to commit myself to any particular variant of the theory in the present context. I will therefore take from the alternative formulations only those elements which appear essential for a functional analysis of basic reading processes. The resultant scheme has features in common with proposals made by Shallice (1981) as the basis for a classification of acquired reading disorders, but this similarity does not imply an acceptance of the theoretical possibilities represented in Shallice's paper.

For the purpose of discussing basic reading functions, it appeared to me to be minimally necessary to postulate central co-operating systems concerned with the representation of meaning and the representation of speech together with a system for the visual analysis and identification of print and writing. I will refer to the first two systems as a 'semantic processor' and a 'phonological processor'. The third system will be referred to as the 'visual (graphemic) processor'. The qualification 'graphemic' is intended to indicate that the processor may be specialised for the handling of print, and is, beyond some peripheral level, functionally distinct from the visual processing required for the analysis and identification of objects (Seymour, 1973; Warren and Morton, 1982). In Figure 2.1 these three components are shown in the form of a simple diagram in which boxes represent complex though specialised information processors and arrows represent pathways for communication between processors.

The following is a preliminary definition of the functions which are presumed to be carried out by the three processors:

Semantic processor
This system is postulated as the basis of 'comprehension' and 'understanding' and as the origin of 'intentions' which may be expressed through speech or action. It is assumed to be involved in the specification of semantic features of verbal concepts, references to objects and the construction of syntactic interpretations.

Phonological processor
This is envisaged as a speech production system which contains a vocabulary store (equivalent to the 'output logogen system' in Morton

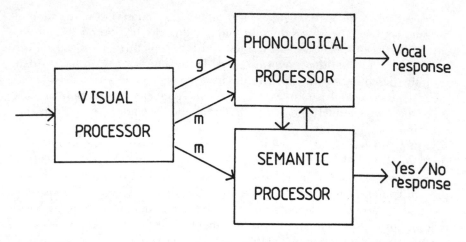

FIGURE 2.1   *Schematic representation of functional model of basic reading processes*

and Patterson's theory), rules of grammatical expression and a phonemic level of speech representation.

Visual (graphemic) processor
This is a system specialised for the analysis of print and handwriting and for the recognition of familiar graphemic forms, including letters, recurring letter groups, free and bound morphemes and words.

In the diagram the arrows represent the flow of information from one processor to another. The analysis of reading functions is primarily concerned with the relationship between the visual processor and the semantic and phonological processors. This relationship is expressed by three arrows, one labelled 'g' and the other two labelled 'm'. The 'g' arrow represents the transmission of sub-lexical graphemic components to the phonological processor, that is the identities of letters, familiar vowel and consonant groupings and possibly syllables or parts of syllables. The 'm' arrows represent the transmission of morphemic information and depend on recognition of whole words or word stems or familiar affixes. The two 'm' arrows imply a distinction between morpheme-based access to semantics and morpheme-based access to phonology.

The model, like that of Morton and Patterson (1980), acknowledges the possibility of three routes by which words may be read. I will refer to these as: (1) the morphemic route to semantics; (2) the morphemic route to phonology; and (3) the grapheme-phoneme translation route.

Morphemic route to semantics
The operation of this route requires the recognition of a word or

morpheme within the visual processor, and the transmission of a signal along the pathway labelled 'm' from the visual processor to the semantic processor. Operations within the semantic processor may control a motor response which indicates comprehension or which expresses the outcome of a judgment. Alternatively, transmission of information from the semantic processor to the phonological processor can result in a selection from the vocabulary store (output logogen) and the production of speech.

Morphemic route to phonology
This route depends on recognition of a word or morpheme in the visual processor and transmission of a signal along pathway 'm' to the phonological processor where an appropriate entry in the vocabulary store (output logogen) can be directly addressed and then produced as a vocal response.

Grapheme-phoneme translation route
Recognition of graphemes and grapheme clusters within the visual processor results in the transmission of signals along pathway 'g' from the visual processor to the phonological processor where entries in a store of phonemic elements can be addressed. These elements may be sequentially organised within the processor and used for direct control over speech production. Alternatively, they may be referred to the vocabulary store (output logogen) and may be helpful in selection of an item from the store.

This formulation leaves open questions about the degree of functional separation of the morphemic route to phonology and the grapheme-phoneme translation route. The two procedures appear to be quite distinct conceptually. However, it is possible that they are functionally interactive. The model is neutral on this point, but allows for interaction in that (1) the products of grapheme-phoneme translation may address vocabulary, and (2) the phonemic store and the vocabulary store are represented as alternative sources of information within the phonological processor.

2.3 Visual processor functions

The visual processor is the one component of the model which is constructed specifically for the purpose of establishing and extending reading skill. I would see it as containing at its highest level a 'recognition space' analogous to the 'visual input logogen' postulated in Morton and Patterson's theory, or the 'word-form system' in Shallice's (1981) account. The function of the visual processor might be seen as one of transforming un-analysed visual data into forms which are recognisable within the space (e.g. abstract visual codes in which letter identities and positions are specified).

The routes labelled 'g' and 'm' from the visual processor to the phonological processor are distinguished from one another in terms of the sizes of the graphemic units they identify. In route 'm', these are relatively large, corresponding to whole words or at least to word stems or familiar affixes. In route 'g' they may be as small as single graphemes or two-to-three letter clusters representing vowels and consonants. Following Shallice (1981) I will argue that this distinction implies the availability of a selective process which is capable of extracting from the abstract representation of the raw input subsets of letter identities of varying size.

I think it might be permissible to refer to a process dealing with multi-letter segments as large as words as being 'wholistic', whereas a process dealing with segments as small as single letters could be called 'analytic'. It would be quite arbitrary to attempt to specify some intermediate unit size which distinguished between wholistic and analytic processing. I therefore propose to use the term 'analytic' to refer to the extreme condition of letter-by-letter processing and the term 'wholistic' to refer to the opposite extreme of whole word processing. The term 'segmental' might be appropriate for the intermediate condition in which letter groups of varying size are handled.

This discussion suggests that the functions of the visual processor might be described in terms of three broadly defined levels which correspond approximately to those proposed by Shallice (1981).

Level of abstract coding
As an initial step, raw visual input is converted into an abstract code which is superordinate to distinctions of type face or handwriting (possibly including the differences between upper and lower case letters). This code specifies letter identities and positions.

Level of parsing and data transfer
A selective process parses the coded array into segments of varying size, possibly making use of categories such as vowel, consonant or syllable, and refers each segment to the recognition space.

Level of recognition
Familiar segments are recognised as morphemes, or as pronounceable vocalic, consonantal or syllabic groupings. Assignment of an identity at this level results in the transmission of an identifying code to the semantic processor or to the phonological processor.

These comments inevitably contain an element of speculation. However, they provide a set of working assumptions which can be used to guide the interpretation of visual processor effects.

2.4 Developmental considerations

A model of the kind described in the previous sections provides a framework within which the cognitive processes of mature readers can be discussed. Such models have proved useful in the analysis of acquired disorders of reading because they lend themselves quite readily to explanations which are stated in terms of the likely effect of a selective impairment of a particular system or route. The model, viewed as a representation of a set of options available to a competent reader, encourages speculations about the kind of performance which might be observed if some of the processes were obliterated or degraded (Marshall and Newcombe, 1973; Shallice, 1981; Patterson, 1982).

The applicability of a model of this general type to an analysis of the acquisition of basic reading skills is more obviously open to question. Developmental theories are often specified in a somewhat different terminology. For example, Bryant and Bradley (1980) speak of the use of a 'phonological strategy' and a 'visual strategy' in reading. Frith (1985) uses the expressions 'logographic strategy' and 'alphabetic strategy' to refer to options for sight word recognition and grapheme-phoneme translation which become available as reading skill develops. A description of development in terms of the availability of strategies lends itself quite readily to a broader theory in which reading acquisition is said to progress through a series of stages, each characterised by the emergence and use of a new strategy (Marsh, Friedman, Welch and Desberg, 1981; Frith, 1985).

The developmental analysis can be assimilated to the information processing framework if it is accepted (1) that a 'strategy' is an information processing concept, and (2) that for a child at any given developmental level there exists a functional model which identifies the processing systems and pathways which are currently available to him. Thus, Frith's logographic and alphabetic strategies can be equated with the operations of the 'm' and 'g' routes and a developmental progression could be represented as a series of models of the type shown in Figure 2.1. One possibility is that all members of this series should be capable of being accommodated within the framework postulated for the mature reader. Reading development could then be said to involve:

(1) the construction of a processing system or sub-system which is present in the adult model but which is absent early in reading development;

(2) an expansion of the resources available to a particular system or sub-system;

(3) strategic variations in the use made of particular systems or sub-systems.

In the model, the phonological processor and the semantic processor are assumed to predate the acquisition of reading skill since a child already possesses a sophisticated knowledge of his world and the uses of spoken language when he enters primary school and embarks on the task of learning to read. The visual (graphemic) processor, on the other hand, is an essential component of the adult model which is absent from the model of a pre-reader, at least in so far as the visual processor is viewed as a graphemic specialist which is functionally distinct from the processor involved in visual object recognition.

The construction of a visual (graphemic) processor is a complex achievement which is fundamental to reading development. In the stage theories of Marsh *et al.* (1981) and Frith (1985) it is considered to begin with the ability to discriminate and recognise words from a limited 'sight vocabulary'. Within the terminology of the information processing model, this could be seen as a matter of determining the features which are useful in discriminating between words and in establishing a mapping between locations in the discrimination space and entries in the semantic processor and in the vocabulary store of the phonological processor. An empirical investigation of this early word learning, reported by Seymour and Elder (1986), suggested that features of word length, salient letter shapes, and letter position might be functional. Beginning readers appeared to possess an episodically stored knowledge of their reading vocabulary and it seemed possible that this was the basis of the route 'm' mapping between the visual processor and the phonological processor. The reaction time to read words was not systematically affected by the number of letters presented. In many instances, severe distortions of word shape were not seriously destructive of accuracy in word reading, although the distortions did generally involve a time cost. These data were obtained from children who were in the process of building up a sight vocabulary of a hundred or more words in the absence of a generalised procedure for grapheme-phoneme translation.

A second developmental process described in the stage theories involves the establishment of grapheme-phoneme correspondences (called the 'alphabetic strategy' by Frith). Gibson, Pick, Osser and Hammond (1962) described this stage as the development of a capability for discrimination of graphemes and grapheme clusters having an invariant relationship with pronunciation. These grapheme clusters were called 'spelling patterns' by Gibson, and were discussed by reference to a syllabic consonant-vowel-consonant (C-V-C) structure as being categorisable as (1) initial consonant spellings, (2) terminal consonant spellings, and (3) vowel spellings. I assume that these categories have to be available phonologically before they can be used as a basis for differentiation of spelling patterns within the graphemic array. This development can be viewed as the emergence of a sub-process within the phonological processor which includes an accessible store of phonemic elements and procedures for ordering and combining discrete phonemes in speech.

The accompanying development within the visual processor involves the establishment of a space for discrimination of graphemes and grapheme clusters, possibly organised in terms of the vowel/consonant and positional categories (Seymour and MacGregor, 1984; Seymour, 1986). The setting up of a rudimentary grapheme-phoneme translation channel (route 'g' to phonology) depends additionally on the establishment of a mapping from the points in the discrimination space onto the phonemic elements stored in the phonological processor.

In the accounts put forward by Marsh *et al.* (1981) and Frith (1985) the word recognition capability is assumed to develop earlier than the grapheme-phoneme translation ability – in Frith's terms, the 'logographic stage' precedes the 'alphabetic stage'. In my view, the models do not take adequate account of the likely impact of teaching methods on the way in which these stages are scheduled. In the class of beginning readers studied by Seymour and Elder (1986), the teacher deliberately concentrated on sight word learning during the first year and delayed the start of phonics instruction until the second year (although some phonics concepts were introduced through writing). Under a regime of this kind it is to be expected that the logographic stage will precede the alphabetic stage. Further, if sound-letter associations are stressed in writing and spelling, then it becomes likely that some children may be shown to be capable of constructing appropriate C-V-C spellings for simple words which they have not been taught to read. This phenomenon of spelling words which cannot be read was noted by Bryant and Bradley (1980) and by Seymour and Elder (1986).

In the present context, the exact schedule of early logographic and alphabetic learning is not critical. The important point is that these two types of learning are required for the establishment of a first approximation to a processing system of the kind suggested in Figure 2.1. I think it is likely that this is normally achieved within the first two to three years at primary school. Hence, the model in Figure 2.1 probably constitutes a reasonable representation of the processing system underlying the reading of children aged 8 and over.

If this view is taken, reading development beyond age 8 is principally a matter of expansion of resources available within a standardised framework. These resources consist in the range of vocabulary discriminated by the visual processor and the size and sophistication of the set of grapheme-phoneme correspondences which has been established.

2.5 Representation of individual differences within the model

In a cognitive analysis of developmental dyslexia the critical questions concern (1) the identification of the elements of a dyslexic processing system which are impaired, and (2) the possibility that subjects will exhibit differing patterns of impairment. The first issue requires a comparison between the processors of dyslexic readers and those of normally competent readers. The second is a matter of contrasting the patterns of impairment shown by different dyslexic subjects.

The information processing model can accommodate individual differences in terms similar to those proposed for the analysis of distinctions between developmental levels. Differences between individuals could arise because:

(1) certain systems or sub-systems were absent for some subjects;
(2) the resources available to particular systems or sub-systems differed between subjects;
(3) subjects differed in their strategic emphasis on the use of particular processing routes.

For any individual reader, it should be possible to construct an information processing model which is descriptive of the configuration he has established, or, alternatively, to represent his configuration within the framework of the standard model.

Cognitive descriptions are interpretations of data which are expressed in the terminology of the information processing system. Initially, therefore, each descriptive statement makes reference to a particular component of the model. At this level, a decision as to whether that component is said to function in an anomalous way depends on a comparison between the relevant experimental data yielded by the dyslexic subject and comparable data obtained from competent readers. A cognitive description consists of a set of statements, each referring to a component of the model, and each containing (1) an evaluative assertion, based on a comparison between the subject's data and the 'normal' data, and (2) a set of interpretative assertions regarding the organisation of a particular locality of the processing system. Just how many such statements are derived depends on how differentiated the model is and how extensive an experimental programme is applied.

The conjunction of these sets of evaluative and interpretative statements defines an overall description of the individual subject's 'information processing configuration'. This can be defined as a set of statements which indicate which elements of the processing system are absent or limited by availability of resources, what strategic biases are present and how particular components are thought to operate.

It is at the level of these configurational descriptions that the question of sub-types arises. Adjudication between the homogeneity, sub-type and heterogeneity proposals depends on judgments regarding the degree of dissimilarity between configurational descriptions which an investigator requires in order to claim that two information processing systems are different from one another. At a somewhat deeper level, there is a question about the manner in which a processing system develops, relating particularly to the degree of independence which may exist between systems and sub-systems. If there is a fixed set of dependencies, such that the development of system B is dependent on the prior development of system A, then an impairment of A will tend always to be accompanied by an impairment of B. If there was a limited number of possible primary impairments, each having a particular set of consequences for development, then each one of these would be likely to be associated with a particular configuration of deficits, and an analysis of dyslexia in terms of sub-types would be favoured. A limiting case of this same proposal is one in which there is a single primary impairment which tends to produce a certain pattern of consequences throughout the system. In such a situation, all dyslexic cases would present similar configurations, and a decision in favour of the homogeneity of dyslexia would be supported.

A further possibility is that a measure of independence exists between systems, such that a primary impairment affects the system within which it is localised while having no necessary consequences for the development of other systems. In this case, a large number of different configurations could occur, depending on which systems were affected and how severely. However, if gradations of severity were categorised, and if the number of processing components entering into the configurational description was limited, such an outcome might be described in terms of a relatively large number of sub-types rather than as a demonstration of heterogeneity.

This discussion poses some additional problems regarding the way in which the term 'dyslexia' is defined and used. In Chapter 1 I argued that, at a level of competence, the term referred simply to the observation that an individual could not accomplish some reading and spelling tasks at a level appropriate for his age. At the cognitive level the term refers either to a particular processing configuration, which is considered to be defective, or to an impairment affecting a particular system or sub-system. A commitment to configurational definitions implies an a priori acceptance of the sub-type hypothesis, i.e. the proposal that there exists a limited number of localised causes which produce characteristic chains of effects. Thus, an expression such as 'developmental phonological dyslexia', as used by Temple and Marshall (1983), is to be taken to refer to a particular processing configuration analogous to that found in cases of acquired phonological dyslexia.

An alternative possibility is that the term 'dyslexia', together with an appropriate qualification, should be used to refer to a disturbance localised in a particular processing system or sub-system. In this usage, 'phonological dyslexia' would be taken to refer to a disturbance affecting the grapheme-to-phoneme translation sub-process within the phonological processor. A 'morphemic dyslexia' would refer to an impairment of route 'm' to phonology or semantics. This approach seems preferable to a usage which allows these terms to refer to complex configurations which carry implications about the states of a number of systems. The more localised reference is consistent with the arguments for adopting a presumption in favour of heterogeneity as a starting point for research. It allows for the possibility of independence in the effects of impairments and gives scope for the description of a wide variety of configurations, ranging from 'pure' cases in which one system is impaired to more complex cases in which a number of systems are affected and the balance of impairments may vary.

2.6 Conclusions

In this chapter I have outlined the properties of an information processing model of basic reading functions which I propose to use as the basis of a cognitive analysis of reading dysfunction in individual cases of developmental dyslexia. The model takes the form of a simple tripartite scheme in which visual, phonological and semantic processors are identified and some aspects of their internal workings and pathways of inter-communication are specified.

If such a model is to be useful in an analysis of dyslexia it is essential that it should be capable of representing differences between subjects which are attributable to their developmental level or the nature of their impairment. I have argued that this can be done by treating the standard model as a framework which defines a set of processing options some of which may be absent or degraded in individual cases.

3 Experimental tasks and factors

3.1 Introduction

The previous chapter outlined some assumptions regarding the manner in which a cognitive method might be applied to the analysis of dyslexic reading. The intention in this and the following chapter is to describe the method in more concrete detail. This involves a consideration of the tasks which appear most appropriate for an investigation of the systems and pathways specified in the model and of the factors which should be varied. The next chapter will discuss some of the technicalities of the research, including the setting up of the experimental procedure on a microcomputer, the conduct of the experiments, and the treatment of the data.

3.2 Experimental tasks

It is convenient to discuss the selection of experimental tasks by reference to the processing routes specified in the model in Figure 2.1. These are the 'm' and 'g' routes from the visual processor to the phonological processor, which are required for reading words aloud, and the 'm' route from the visual processor to the semantic processor, which is involved in comprehension. Two types of task were needed to assess these routes, which I shall refer to as 'vocalisation tasks' and 'decision tasks'. In the vocalisation tasks the subject was presented with single visual words and non-words and was asked to read them aloud. Measures of vocal reaction time (VRT), accuracy and error type were taken. The decision tasks involved judgments about visual, lexical or semantic properties of a stimulus which were signalled by a Yes or No key-press response. Measures of accuracy and Yes/No reaction time (RT) were recorded.

Vocalisation tasks

According to the model in Figure 2.1 the task of reading aloud visually presented words depends on the analysis and recognition of the item within the visual (graphemic) processor and the retrieval of a naming response from a vocabulary store located within the phonological processor (route 'm' to phonology). The model allows that response retrieval may be assisted by concurrent semantic processing or by concurrent grapheme-phoneme translation. These processes were tested by experiments in which the subjects were presented with isolated words on a screen and were asked to read them out aloud as rapidly and as accurately as possible.

The second route to phonology, labelled route 'g' in Figure 2.1, is assumed to involve the transmission of identities of graphemes to the phonological processor where phonemic elements can be retrieved from a store and assembled for production as speech. The assumption was made that the task of reading aloud unfamiliar non-words was likely to engage this translation process. I am aware that this proposal might be taken to imply a rejection of the view, ably expressd by Henderson (1982), that non-word reading could be achieved by operations on the pronunciations of stored vocabulary. However, I would regard such theories primarily as variants on specific proposals as to how the translation process might work, or, more exactly, what sources of information it might draw on. I will, therefore, use the non-word reading task as a procedure for testing route 'g' to phonology, though without a wish to imply a commitment to any particular theory of the translation process, or any degree of separation or merging of the 'm' and 'g' pathways.

Visual matching tasks

Posner and Mitchell (1967) introduced the idea of levels at which subjects might be instructed to make 'same'-'different' judgments and distinguished between a level of physical identity and higher levels of name or rule (semantic) identity. At the physical identity level the subject is instructed to respond 'same' to items which are visually identical. The experimental evidence suggests that these judgments are based on visual data. I will make the assumption that physical identity matching involves a decision about data which are arrayed within the visual processor component of Figure 2.1.

Two types of visual matching task were used in the assessment of visual processor functions. I will refer to these as the 'identity matching task' and the 'array matching task'.

The identity matching task was a variant of Posner and Mitchell's procedure which was introduced by Beller (1970). Posner and Mitchell used pairs of letters or digits in their experiments, but Beller used larger arrays of varying size. He found that decisions that arrays of 2, 4 or 8 letters contained only 'same' items were made by a parallel process, that is with a reaction time which was not affected by the number of letters on the display. Thus, his adult subjects were able to indicate that

AA   AAAA   AAAAAAAA

were 'same' displays with equivalent reaction times. I will make the assumption that the data on which such decisions are based are formed early on in the operations of the visual processor, possibly at a level of feature extraction which directly precedes, or is coincidental with, the formation of an input code representing letter identities and positions. If these assumptions are well-founded, then it should be possible to use the identity matching task as a procedure for assessing the efficiency of a preliminary level of operation within the visual processor.

The second type of visual matching task, referred to as the array matching task, involved the simultaneous presentation of two letter arrays, each containing 5 letters, positioned one above the other. The subject was instructed to classify the display as 'same' if the arrays contained the same letters in the same positions, and as 'different' if there were any positions containing different letters. On 'different' trials all letters could be different, or there might be only a single difference which varied in position, viz.:

CXQJR   CXQJR   CXQJR   CXQJR
CXQJR   MBZPN   CYQJR   CXQBR

The assumption was made that the comparison of pairs of arrays was likely to engage the analytic functions of the visual processor and thus to provide information relating to the parsing level of the processor.

Lexical and semantic decision tasks

There were two other types of decision task which were intended to tap somewhat higher levels of processing, involving word recognition and access to semantics. The 'lexical decision task' is a widely used procedure in which the subject is presented with a mixed list of words and non-words under instruction to make a Yes response to words and a No response to non-words. The earliest point at which a positive decision could be taken is the morpheme recognition level of the visual processor, although it is possible that the decision is in practice based on retrieval of semantic information or some other higher level code. If the parsing level of the visual processor contains information about orthographic structure, then it

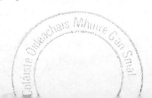

might be possible for illegal non-words, such as LTISPR, to be rejected at that level. Thus, it is assumed that the lexical decision task has the potential for providing information about orthographic coding within the visual processor as well as about the level of word recognition and semantic access.

The second task was a 'semantic decision task'. This was also a variant of a standard experimental procedure in which the subject is presented with the name of a category of objects followed by the name of an instance which he must classify by a Yes response if it is a member of the named category and by a No response if it is not, e.g.

$$\text{FURNITURE} \ldots \text{table} \rightarrow \text{Yes}$$
$$\text{FURNITURE} \ldots \text{tulip} \rightarrow \text{No}$$

It was assumed that this task requires access to semantic information (route 'm' from the visual processor to the semantic processor) and the application of comparison and decision procedures to the semantic codes which have been retrieved.

3.3 Factor variations in the word reading tasks

Fundamental to the method of cognitive psychology is the notion that the components of an information processing system can be investigated by a procedure which involves systematic variations in factors which are thought to exert a selective influence on a particular process. The experimental method involves observations of the effects of these variations on measurable indicators, such as the reaction time or the accuracy or form of the response, and the effects are then treated as a basis for inferences about properties of the processing system. In this and the following sections I will explain what factors were varied within each task, what process or route they were considered to influence, and the interpretations of the effects which were favoured.

The task of reading aloud known words was intended as a measure of the functioning of route 'm' to phonology. Certain factor variations were imposed on this task with the aim of obtaining information about (1) visual processor functions underlying vocalisation of words, (2) effects of familiarity on word reading, and (3) the possible involvement of semantic processing or grapheme-phoneme translation in the retrieval of a vocal response to a word.

Two sets of factors were considered relevant to the analysis of the visual processor functions. These were (1) word length, and (2) the format in which a word was presented.

Word length

The words presented to the subjects varied in length, that is in the number of letters they contained. It was considered that this factor varied the load imposed on the parsing level of the visual processor. In some accounts of word recognition it is proposed that words are parsed wholistically, allowing either for the simultaneous reference of all component letters to the recognition space or for the extraction of identifying features in parallel. If parsing involves no systematic serial component, then it is to be expected that variations in word length will not be associated with variations in reading reaction time. If, on the other hand, parsing is typically analytic (focused on single letters) or segmental (focused on letter groups), and there is a serial element in the transfer of these elements to the recognition space, then it is to be expected that reading reaction time will increase as a function of the number of letters contained in a word. If this increase approximates a linear function, then the slope of the function (the amount by which the reaction time increases for each additional letter on the display) may conveniently be used as an index of the rate of functioning of the parsing level of the visual processor.

Format distortion

In the main set of experiments words were presented in normal format, that is as a horizontal array of letters ordered from left to right. Other experiments incorporated a factor of format distortion under which words were presented normally or with a zigzag or vertical arrangement of letters, e.g.

		T
TABLE	T B E	A
	A L	B
		L
		E

The assumption was made that these spatial distortions were likely to impose a load on visual processor functions. The exact form of this load depends on the manner in which the parsing and recognition processes operate, and particularly on the extent to which the recognition space is tuned to accept only inputs which have a standard spatial structure. It is, for example, possible that the recognition space is tuned to accept arrays which include a coding of horizontal position on a left-right axis. The distortions violate these requirements and it might therefore be necessary for the processor to spend some time 'normalising' the spatial code before recognition could occur. In order to gain information on this point, the format variations were always combined with a length variation. It was expected that a recoding operation which restructured the spatial relations between letters or letter groups in a serial manner would produce an interaction between word length and format distortion, such that length effects appeared to be exaggerated when distorted words were read. A result of this kind is typically obtained when skilled adult readers are asked to respond to normal and distorted words. A length effect of about 10 ms/letter observed for the reading of normally formatted words may rise to about 100 ms/letter when vertically distorted words are read. This effect of length on the reading of distortions defines the rate at which the processor can operate when required to proceed in a serial mode.

The other factors which were incorporated into the experiments were intended to assess the impact of familiarity on the operation of route 'm' to phonology, and also the extent of co-operative involvement of grapheme-phoneme translation and semantic processing. The familiarity effect was assessed by varying the normative frequency of usage of the words. A variation in spelling-to-sound regularity was used to assess the contribution of the grapheme-phoneme translation process. The contribution of the semantic processor was tested by varying part of speech and concreteness of meaning.

Word frequency

The frequencies with which words occur in large samples of text have been quantified in published word counts (Thorndike and Lorge, 1944; Kucera and Francis, 1967). This factor was varied by drawing samples of words from the A and AA categories in the Thorndike-Lorge count and samples with frequencies of 30 occurrences per million or fewer. These samples were respectively designated as 'high frequency words' and 'low frequency words'. It was assumed that if the pathway 'm' from the visual processor to the phonological processor was biased by frequency of occurrence then words of high frequency would be read faster or more accurately than words of low frequency. The occurrence of a 'word frequency effect' was then treated as an indication of an involvement of route 'm' in reading aloud.

Spelling-to-sound regularity

As was noted earlier, Gibson proposed that the perceptual basis of grapheme-phoneme correspondence learning might be the abstraction of letter groups, called spelling patterns, which stood in an invariant relation to sound. Many English words are built up from these consonant and vowel spelling patterns and may be said to contain regular spelling-to-sound correspondences. Other words contain spelling patterns which are inconsistent in correspondence, or which are frankly exceptional. These may be referred to as 'irregular words', although it is probably true that differing degrees of irregularity are possible (Shallice, Warrington and McCarthy, 1983). A list of high and low frequency words was constructed which contained words considered to embody consistent or regular correspondences and words considered to be inconsistent or irregular. The list has been reproduced in Appendix 1. The assumption was made that processing via the grapheme-phoneme translation channel (route 'g' to phonology) would be adversely affected by spelling-to-sound irregularity. This is because the translation channel, by interpreting the input in terms of standard correspondences, is likely to produce an incorrect phonological representation for an irregular word. This may result in a conflict of output phonologies, giving rise to a delay of reaction, or to the production of an incorrect response, which will sometimes be a 'regularisation' (e.g. 'shoe' pronounced as 'show'). Hence, the occurrence of a 'regularity effect' will be taken as an indication that some grapheme-phoneme processing is involved in the retrieval of a response to a word. In the terms of the model, this means that the operation of route 'm' to phonology can be supported by concurrent activity in route 'g'.

Concreteness and form class

These semantic/syntactic dimensions were introduced in order to test for the involvement of semantic processing during word retrieval. The reading of 'deep dyslexic' patients has been shown to be impaired for words of abstract meaning and for words having a primarily syntactic function (Shallice and Warrington, 1975). It is probable that these patients read via the semantic processor and that their performance indicates a restriction on the capacity of this system to generate speech for abstract or grammatical meanings. If this is a general property of the relationship between the semantic processor and the phonological processor, then it should follow that a reliance on semantic processing as a support for word retrieval will result in concreteness or form class effects. To test for these influences a second word list was compiled which included a set of high frequency function words, and sets of high and low frequency content words stratified into concrete and abstract subsets. Concreteness was defined by reference to the norms published by Paivio, Yuille and Madigan (1968). The list appears in Appendix 1.

3.4 Factor variations in the non-word reading task

The non-word reading task was employed as a procedure for assessing the grapheme-phoneme translation route from the visual processor to the phonological processor. The contrast between performance on this task and performance on the word reading task may be referred to as the 'lexicality effect' (the difference in accuracy or reaction time between word reading and non-word reading). This effect is particularly important in the analysis of reading disability, since a large divergence between word and non-word reading has been taken to imply a selective deficit in the translation process.

   The non-word reading experiments incorporated the visual processor variations already mentioned (non-word length and format distortion) together with other factors considered to relate to the translation process. These included (1) the graphemic complexity of the vowel structures contained in the non-words, (2) the consistency of the lexical environment from which the non-word was sampled, and (3) whether or not the non-word, when pronounced, was a homophone of an English word.

Non-word length

The non-words presented for reading aloud varied in the number of letters they contained. It has already been suggested that route 'g' to phonology may operate by identifying phonologically significant grapheme clusters within the visual processor. This requires analytic or segmental parsing. If the parser transfers data serially to the grapheme recognition space it is expected that reaction time to read non-words will be sensitive to non-word length. The translation process is also assumed to involve the retrieval of phonemic elements from a store and their assembly for pronunciation. A limitation on the rate at which data were handled might also arise at this phonological stage. In this case, the processing rate for non-words, expressed in milliseconds per letter, could be taken as an index of graphemic parsing or phonemic retrieval and assembly, whichever was the slower.

Format distortion

The interpretation of effects of format distortion on non-word reading is similar to that proposed for word reading. Distortion is expected to impose an additional load on the visual processor and to force the adoption of a serial analytic processing mode. The effect, defined in terms of processing time per letter, is likely to be larger for non-words than for words, because the processor may be subject to the impact of distortion combined with existing limitations on the rate at which information can be transferred during grapheme-phoneme translation.

Graphemic complexity

The vowel spelling patterns contained in the non-words were classified as simple (one grapheme only) or as complex (more than one grapheme). An effect of this variable was taken as an indication of a limitation on the scope of the grapheme recognition space or its capacity to address the phonemic store.

Non-word homophony

A non-word may be a written neologism which does not represent the sound of any English word or may be a homophone of a known word (e.g. skule). This distinction between homophones and non-homophones was built into some of the non-word lists. The assumption was made that an effect of non-word homophony on reading accuracy or reaction time would indicate that output from the grapheme-phoneme translator was referred to the vocabulary store (output logogen) in order to assist response production. This proposal entails a further differentiation within the phonological processor in Figure 2.1. It is suggested that route 'g' to phonology generates as output a phonemic code which may directly control speech production or which may be used as an input to the vocabulary store. If this input matches a stored item fairly directly, then that item may be produced as a response. Thus, a homophony effect is taken as an indication of a tendency to lexicalise output from the grapheme-phoneme translation channel. Appendix 2 contains a non-word list in which the factor of homophony is combined with a variation in vowel complexity.

Lexical environment

In his discussion of phonological retrieval in reading Glushko (1979) argued that the time to read a word was affected by the consistency of its lexical environment. This was defined mainly by reference to the way in which the vowel was pronounced when followed by a given terminal consonant group. For example, the vowel 'ea' followed by the consonant 'd' is inconsistent because it is pronounced one way in words like 'bead' and another in words like 'head'. Glushko presented data to suggest that non-words containing ambiguous segments of this kind (e.g. 'yead') were also subject to a time penalty in speeded naming tasks. In order to examine these effects, the environments for the simple vowels in combination with 56 initial consonant groups and 75 terminal groups were plotted and the vowel + consonant groups which were inconsistent in pronunciation were identified. A non-word list which contained items from consistent and inconsistent environments involving standard and non-standard vowel pronunciation was constructed. Table 3.1 gives the frequencies of lexicalised and non-lexicalised reponses made by adult subjects when reading the items from this list (Maccabe, 1984). It can be seen that the frequency of lexicalised pronunciations approached 50 per cent for items drawn from consistently irregular environments but was considerably lower in the other cases. This list proved useful in determining whether or not subjects made use of vowel + terminal consonant structures when assigning pronunciation to non-words. For example, words ending in '-alk' are pronounced /ɔːk/ rather than /ælk/.

TABLE 3.1   *Frequencies of regular and 'lexicalised' vowel pronunciations in responses to non-words from consistent and inconsistent environments by adult subjects (data from Maccabe, 1984)*

| | Consistent environment | | Inconsistent environment | | |
	Regular pronunciation	Irregular pronunciation	Regular bias	Irregular bias	Overall
Regular vowel pronunciation	333	179	136	116	764
'Lexicalised' vowel pronunciation	–	166	3	43	212
Per cent use of lexical correspondence		48.12	2.16	27.04	21.72

If a non-word, such as 'dalk', is pronounced to rhyme with 'walk' this suggests that the correspondence '-alk' → /ɔːk/ has been used (Patterson and Morton, 1985), or, alternatively, that the lexical environment containing words with this orthographic ending has been consulted (Henderson, 1982). This list also appears in Appendix 2.

3.5 Factor variations in the matching and decision tasks

As was mentioned in Section 3.2, two types of visual matching task were used as a procedure for assessing the efficiency of the visual processor. The 'identity matching task' involved simple physical judgments about arrays of letters and was considered to tap processing at a relatively early stage. The array matching task required comparison between two arrays of letters and was thought to involve a more analytic procedure, possibly located at the level of the parser.

Identity matching

The factors varied in the identity matching task were (1) the response required (Yes or No), (2) the size of the letter array (3, 7 or 11 letters), and (3) the number of different letters present on No trials (all or one only). The location of the single difference varied between the left, central and right-hand regions of the display. The factor of principal interest was the array size. The absence of an effect of the number of letters presented was taken as an indication that parallel processing was possible at the level at which identity was detected.

In addition to the standard experiment, two further identity matching experiments were set up. One of these incorporated a variation in the format of presentation (normal, zigzag or vertical). The second varied the orientation of the letters (normal or mirror image).

Array matching

The factors varied in the array matching task included one psycholinguistic variable, the legality of the letter sequences. Legality was varied by contrasting randomly chosen letter sequences with sequences constructed from appropriately positioned consonant and vowel spelling patterns, e.g.

SLART	SLART	RTBLJ	RTBLJ
SLART	SPART	RTBLJ	RZBLJ

Previous research by Chambers and Forster (1975) and others has indicated that skilled adult readers typically match legal arrays faster than illegal arrays, especially on Yes trials. It was assumed that a 'legality effect' of this kind implied that information about English orthographic structure had been internalised within the visual processor and was available to the matching operation.

The other factors which were varied were: (1) the response required (Yes or No), (2) the number of differences (all or one), and (3) the position of the single difference (1 to 5). Array size was fixed at 5 letters. It was assumed that if comparison is a serial self-terminating procedure which progresses from left to right across the array, then No reaction time will increase as a function of the position of the single difference, and the slope of this function can be taken as an index of the rate at which the comparison process operates. The self-terminating model also predicts that 'all different' displays should be classified faster than 'single difference' displays and that Yes responses should be slower than No responses.

The standard array matching experiment was supplemented by two additional studies, one involving a format variation (horizontal arrays versus vertical arrays), and the other a variation in letter orientation (normal versus mirror image letters).

Lexical decisions

In the lexical decision task subjects were asked to indicate, by a Yes or No key-press response, whether the item on the display was a known word or a non-word. Three manipulations were included which were thought to be selectively related to the visual processor functions: (1) word and non-word length, (2) the format of presentation, and (3) the orthographic legality of the non-words. There was also a variation in the frequency of occurrence of the word stimuli.

In the standard experiment, words of high and low frequency and legal and illegal non-words were presented in standard format, e.g.

TABLE   CRADLE   SLART   RTBSL

It was considered that a 'frequency effect' on the latency or accuracy of responses to words was indicative of a bias located within the morpheme recognition space of the visual processor or in route 'm' to the semantic processor. A 'legality effect' on responses to non-words was expected to take the form of faster and more accurate rejection of the illegal items. The words and non-words also varied in length. It was considered that the presence or absence of a length effect would be indicative of the type of parsing operation (analytic, segmental or wholistic) involved in the classification of words and legal or illegal non-words when vocalisation was not required.

An additional experiment was constructed in which variations in frequency, legality and length were combined with distortions of format (normal, zigzag or vertical presentation). This procedure was used to assess the effects of imposition of a load on the visual processor in a situation in which processing was oriented towards the semantic processor rather than the phonological processor. The slope of the function relating word length to reaction time was treated as an index of the rate at which the visual processor could operate in analytic mode when resolving distortions for the purpose of morpheme recognition. If illegal non-words can be detected at an earlier level of the visual processor, and hence do not require to be normalised, then length and distortion effects should be relatively slight for these items.

Semantic decisions

In the semantic decision task the subject responded to names of object classes by indicating with a Yes or No key-press response whether or not they were members of a specified superordinate class. It was considered that this task assessed the operation of route 'm' to semantics. Previous investigations of adult subjects by Smith, Shoben and Rips (1974) and others have indicated that the efficiency of semantic decisions is influenced by the semantic relationship existing between the category names and the items used as test instances. Positive instances may vary in their 'typicality' or goodness of fit to the category (Rosch, 1975). For example, 'chair' is a good example of the category of 'furniture', whereas 'rug' is an atypical or marginal instance. Negative instances may be drawn from a category which is semantically close to the target category or from one which is relatively remote from it. Thus, given the category 'tree', 'tulip' could be regarded as a close negative, and 'hammer' as a distant negative. A general finding has been that reaction times are delayed when subjects make positive decisions about atypical instances or negative decisions about instances from related categories. These factors of typicality and relatedness were built into the semantic decision experiment. It was assumed that a 'typicality effect' reflected a bias in the process of accessing semantic information, and that a 'negative relatedness effect' indexed a process of semantic comparison.

The semantic decision experiments also incorporated variations in word length and in the format of presentation. The effects of these factors were treated as indicators of visual processor operations underlying the operation of route 'm' to semantics.

3.6 Mapping of tasks and factors onto processing model

As developed here the 'cognitive method' involves (1) the specification of a functionally defined modular information processing model, (2) the identification of a set of tasks which engage the resources of the processors and the pathways postulated in the model, and (3) the variation, within the context of the tasks, of factors which are thought likely to exert a selective influence on the activities of particular processors or pathways.

In order to make the mapping of the tasks and factors onto the model explicit, Figure 3.1 reproduces the tripartite scheme from Figure 2.1 with the superimposition of the pathways thought to be involved in the tasks of vocalising words and non-words, visual matching and making lexical and semantic decisions. The figure includes the differentiation within the processors suggested by the discussion of factor effects and also indicates the presumed locus of each of the factor variations.

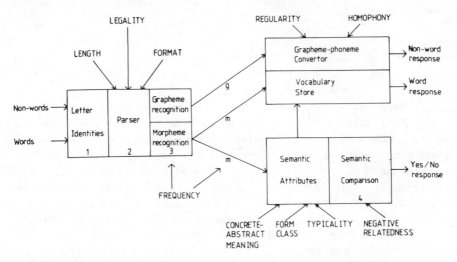

FIGURE 3.1   *Mapping of tasks and factors onto the processing model. Word vocalisation involves route 'm' to the phonological processor. Non-word vocalisation involves route 'g'. The decision tasks engage the visual processor and the semantic processor, with the locus of decision being (1) for identity matching, (2) for array matching, (3) for lexical decisions, and (4) for semantic decisions. The locus of influence of the frequency factor is assumed to be diffuse, including the morpheme recognition space and the 'm' routes*

In discussing the experimental variables it is convenient to make a distinction between 'psycholinguistic factors' and 'processing factors'. In general, the processing factors include manpulations of display size and format which are considered to affect visual processor functions. The psycholinguistic factors are properties of linguistic stimuli which are assumed to have been internalised by literate language users. These include orthographic legality, which is an influence on the visual processor, word frequency, which is a property of the morphemic pathways, spelling-to-sound regularity and homophony which affect the phonological processor, and form class, concreteness of meaning, typicality and relatedness, which are influences on the semantic processor.

4 Methods and procedures

4.1 Introduction

The application of the cognitive method involves the administration, to the individual members of a subject sample, of a series of experiments which embody the task and factor variations considered to be relevant to an investigation of the processing model which is being used as a framework for the research. For present purposes, an 'experiment' will be defined as an episode in which a task instruction is given and a series of displays is presented under conditions which permit the timing of reactions and the recording of the accuracy and characteristics of the responses.

This chapter will give details of the experiments which were administered in the course of the cognitive assessment of reading functions. It will also explain how the procedure was set up on a microprocessor as well as providing information about the practicalities of running the experiments and recording and analysing the results.

4.2 Main set of experiments

The experimental series consisted of a 'core' set of experiments which were completed by all subjects together with some additional studies which were undertaken by most, but not all, of the members of the dyslexic sample.

Table 4.1 identifies the full set of experiments, and gives, for each one, information about the task requirements, the factors which were varied and the number of trials which were involved. The experiments have been grouped according to the processing domain (route 'm' to phonology, route 'g' to phonology, route 'm' to semantics, the visual processor) which they were designed to test.

TABLE 4.1 *Summary of the experimental procedure in which tasks have been grouped according to the processing domain considered to be under test. There were some further replications of the lexical decision and visual matching tasks which are not shown in the table. The main experiments, taken by all subjects, are marked with an asterisk*

Functions	Task	Description	Number	Factors	Trials
Route 'm' to phonology	Vocalisation of words	Read aloud words	1*	Word frequency (H,L)[1] Length (3-7 letters) Abstract-concrete meaning Syntactic function	126
			2*	Word frequency (H,L)[1] Length (3-6 letters) Spelling-to-sound regularity	112
			3*	Word frequency (H,L)[1] Length (3-7 letters) Format (normal, zigzag, vertical)	90
Route 'g' to phonology	Vocalisation of non-words	Read aloud non-words	4	Word frequency (H,L)[1] Length (3-6 letters) Lexicality (word, non-word)	112
			5	Non-word length (3-6 letters)	60
			6*	Non-word length (3-7 letters) Homophony Vowel complexity	120
			7*	Homophony Non-word length (3-7 letters) Format (normal, zigzag, vertical)	90
			8	Non-word length (4-6 letters) Lexical environment	114
Route 'm' to semantics	Semantic categorisation	Press Yes key if word is a member of a specified category, otherwise No key	9*	Typicality of positive instances Relatedness of negative instances Word length (3-8 letters)	120

Functions	Task	Description	Number	Factors	Trials
			10*	Typicality Word length (3-8 letters) Format (normal, zigzag, vertical)	144
	Lexical decision	Press Yes key if item on display is a word, otherwise No key	11*	Word frequency (H,L)[1] Non-word legality Word and non-word length (3-6 letters)	120
			12*	Word frequency (H,L)[1] Non-word legality Word and non-word length (3-7 letters) Format (normal, zigzag, vertical)	180
Visual processor	Identity matching	Press Yes key if all letters on display are 'same', otherwise No key	13*	Display size (3-11 letters) Number of differences Position of single difference	120
			14	Display size (3-11 letters) Format (normal, zigzag, vertical) Position of difference	162
	Array matching	Press Yes key if two 5-letter arrays contain same letters in same positions, otherwise No key	15*	Orthographic legality Position of difference 100	
			16	Format (horizontal vertical) Position of difference	120

1 High frequency words (H) were sampled from the AA and A sets of the Thorndike and Lorge (1944) word count. Low frequency words were sampled from the range below 30 per million, with a mean of about 12 per million.

4.3 Apparatus

The experimental procedure was automated on an Apple II micro-computer. The machine contained 48K RAM and was linked to dual disk drives, a 22 cm × 17 cm green screen monitor, and a printer. A Mountain Hardware Clock/Calendar card was fitted in Slot 4. A voice-operated switch and two microswitches, designated 'Yes' and 'No', were connected to the computer via the games I/O channel.

Interval timing and reaction timing were carried out by assembly language routines based on interrupts generated at 1 ms intervals by the clock. Timing of a delay was achieved by entering the desired interval into two memory locations and calling a procedure which enabled interrupts. An interrupt handler routine subtracted 1 from the memory locations each millisecond. A check for expiry of the interval was made by a second routine which disabled interrupts and returned control to the host program when zero values were detected.

In the case of reaction timing the interrupt handler added 1 to the contents of two memory locations each millisecond while the program repeatedly checked the registers on the games I/O channel for an indication that a switch had closed. A location was set to 0 when testing the Yes switch and to 1 when testing the No switch. Detection of a switch closure caused disabling of interrupts and returned control to the host program which recovered the value of the reaction time and the number of the switch which had been pressed.

The switching on and off of displays was achieved using the Apple 'soft switch' locations. Reference to one location had the effect of switching output to the screen from the computer's graphics memory to its text memory. Reference to a second location had the opposite effect of switching output from text to high resolution graphics. In most of the experiments displays were printed into the text memory while the computer was switched to a blank graphics screen. The display was made visible and timing was started when the text soft switch was thrown.

This procedure gives precise reaction time measurements and also allows a complex display to be built up and then switched on and off abruptly. A small error in timing will occur because the exact onset of the display is contingent on the position of the raster scan of the monitor screen at the instant when the switch is operated. This error can be corrected by fitting a circuit which detects the resetting of the scan and makes the start of reaction timing contingent on this. However, since the error was small relative to the sizes of the effects under investigation and should in any case be randomly distributed across experimental conditions, it was not considered necessary to insist on this additional precision in the present investigation.

4.4 Construction of experiments

The experiments all involved the presentation of a sequence of stimuli in a randomised order. Presentation was by means of a 'display program' which presented targets on the screen, recorded reaction times and responses and permitted the experimenter to type in information about errors. The display program required a 'vocabulary file' and a 'sequence file' to operate.

The 'vocabulary file' was a list of linguistic stimuli organised according to relevant psycholinguistic dimensions. For example, one of the lists in Appendix 1 contains words of high and low frequency, regular and irregular spelling, and length 3, 4, 5 or 6 letters. This gives a $2 \times 2 \times 4$ structure, containing 16 sub-categories of items. In the experiment, 7 items were assigned to each sub-category, making a total of 112 items. A program was written which allowed for the entry and editing of these lists and their placement as text files on floppy disk.

The display program required a second file which controlled the sequence in which items were presented. This is referred to as the 'sequence file' and contained a series of strings each specifying the number of the vocabulary item which should be presented and a code which identified its sub-category and, if necessary, indicated the format in which it should be displayed. The sequence file was made up by a randomiser program which took as input a file specifying the structure of the list, including (1) its length, (2) the number of sub-categories into which it was divided, (3) the numeric range corresponding to each sub-category, and (4) a code by which the sub-category could be identified.

In the experiments in which format distortion was combined with the psycholinguistic and length factors, an additional procedure was introduced which assigned formats at random within each sub-category of the list. Thus, if there were three formats (normal, zigzag and vertical), and 15 items per sub-category, the program would randomly assign 5 items to each format and would mark their entries in the sequence list with a code which was recognisable to the display program.

The sequence-maker program was run prior to each experimental session, so that each subject encountered a new randomisation of the list and a new assignment of formats.

4.5 Conduct of experiments

The experiments were run using a 'display program' into which the appropriate vocabulary file and sequence file had been loaded. The subject was given an explanation of the task followed by a series of between 12 and 20 practice trials after which the main experiment began. The experiment usually consisted of a sequence of a 100 or so 'trials' each involving the presentation of a stimulus and the recording of a reaction time and response. An array of 5 asterisks appeared at the centre of the screen for 500 ms followed after a blank interval of 1500 ms by the target. Displays were formed using the standard Apple upper case character set. The target remained in view until the computer detected a switch closure. The experimenter then indicated on the keyboard whether the response had been correct, a technical failure (e.g. of the voice switch) or an error. In the vocalisation experiments, a representation of the error response was typed in. The program made provision for the replacement of trials which had been lost on account of technical failures.

On each trial the display program obtained the next code from the sequence list and isolated the number of the vocabulary item and, if applicable, a code specifying the format of presentation. The vocabulary item was then retrieved, reformatted if necessary and printed in the text memory during the blank interval between the asterisks and the switching on of the display. In the semantic decision experiments the asterisks were replaced by presentation of the category name for 2000 ms.

The experimenter monitored the subject's response and classified it on the keyboard. The program then advanced to the next trial. If the program encountered a rest code the subject was instructed to take a break and an Apple housekeeping operation was initiated. This was done in order to prevent the computer from interrupting the experiments in an uncontrolled manner. When the program encountered a terminator code a message of gratitude was displayed followed by options to print the raw data and to save the record of the experiment on the disk. This record contained the identifying codes and reaction times of each correct and incorrect trial together with a representation of each error response.

4.6 Treatment of reaction time data

Reaction time measurements are the most sensitive of the indicators employed in cognitive research. Their critical role in the analysis of cognitive functions is based on the assumptions (1) that cognitive processes require measurable intervals of time for their operations, and (2) that the time taken up by a cognitive process can be altered by variations in the levels of psycholinguistic and processing factors. The effect of a variation on the reaction time often provides the essential datum for interpretative statements about the characteristics of particular processes. In the present context, reaction times were interpreted in two distinct ways: (1) the overall level of the reaction time in the performance of a particular task was treated as an index of the efficiency of each of the major pathways postulated in the information processing model; and (2) the effects of the psycholinguistic and processing factor variations were interpreted as indicators of the more detailed characteristics of particular systems or pathways. These two uses can be referred to as the evaluative and the interpretative treatments of the reaction time.

Evaluative treatment of reaction time

The reaction times collected from a subject during one or more experiments formed a distribution of values falling within a certain range and open to description in terms of measures of central tendency and dispersion such as the mean and standard deviation. An estimate of the values of these statistics which could be considered indicative of normally efficient functioning was obtained by applying the main set of experiments to the individual members of a sample of competent readers (see Chapter 5). A subject producing values which lay outside these estimates was considered to provide evidence of inefficiency within the processing systems and routes considered to be involved in the performance of the task.

Although the standard deviation provides a general index of the spread of a reaction time distribution, it does not distinguish between cases where the distribution is approximately normal in shape, though with wide dispersion, and cases where a distribution of faster times is accompanied by a long tail of slower responses. In order to examine this aspect of the data the reaction time distributions were plotted in the form of frequency polygons. An interval of 250 ms was used and a range up to 6000 ms. The data typically yielded an approximation to one of the idealised forms shown in Figure 4.1. A distribution of Type A is located at the fast end of the reaction time scale and the times all fall within a small number of adjacent categories. This type of distribution is characteristic of efficient functioning. In a Type B distribution, a majority of items fall within adjacent categories at the fast end of the scale but there is in addition a tail of slower responses. The occurrence of these occasional slow reactions was taken to be indicative of a minor degree of inefficiency in the underlying process. Type C distributions are characteristic of severely impaired functions. These distributions include no preponderance of fast times and often approximate a rectangular distribution with very wide dispersion.

Reaction time effects

The second use of the reaction time was as a basis for inferences about processing characteristics of individual subjects. Such inferences depend on a demonstration that psycholinguistic or processing factor variations produce a reliable effect on reaction time levels. In general, effects were tested by applying a t-test to compare two reaction time distributions. For

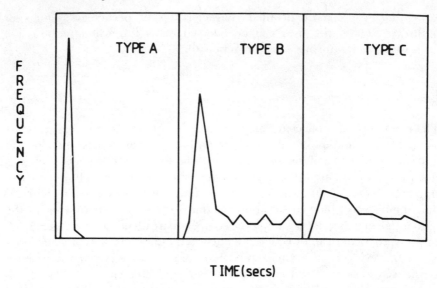

FIGURE 4.1   *Idealised forms of Type A, Type B and Type C reaction time distributions*

example, a 'frequency effect' was said to be present if a t-test comparing the distributions of reaction times to read high frequency words and low frequency words yielded a value of *t* which was significant at $p < 0.05$ or better. In most instances the expected direction of the effect could be specified in advance and the use of probability values for one-tailed tests was considered appropriate.

Where a subject had produced a reaction time distribution of Type B, that is one containing a preponderance of fast times plus a tail of slower times, the data were analysed both with the full set of reaction times and with the outlying responses removed. Occasions when this practice made a difference to the conclusions regarding the significance of effects will be mentioned in the discussions of individual cases.

Length and position effects

The effects of word and non-word length were analysed by calculating the regression of reaction time on the length variable and expressing the outcome as the intercept and slope parameters of the line of best fit (as determined by the least squares procedure). Thus,

$$RT = A + B(L) \text{ ms}$$

where L is the word length in letters, A is the zero intercept and B is the slope. The value of B was treated as an index of the 'rate of processing'. If, for example, the obtained values for the length effects were $A = 500$ ms and $B = 100$ ms, then it was concluded that the function in question operated at a rate of 100 ms per letter. The linearity of the relation between reaction time and word length was assessed by application of an F-test. If this test was significant at $p < 0.05$ or better, then it was concluded that reaction time was related to word length by an approximation to a linear function and this was taken as an indication of the possible involvement of a serial process.

Position of difference effects in the array matching task were analysed in a similar way. Reaction time was expressed as a function of the left-to-right position of the single different letter and the linearity of the function was tested by an F-test. A significant linear trend was taken as evidence for the involvement of a serial self-terminating process operating in a left-to-right direction across the arrays.

4.7 Treatment of error data

The second main indicator of cognitive functioning is the accuracy of response assessed relative to a criterion of adequacy implicit in the task instructions given to the subject. This indicator can be treated evaluatively and interpretatively, and the interpretation can be based on a simple evaluation of accuracy or on a consideration of qualitative aspects of the error. These qualitative aspects bear principally on the nature of the relationship existing between the target and the error response. This can be represented in the form of a classification of relationships or by some more formal procedure of structural analysis and comparison.

Evaluative treatment of errors

The evaluative use of the accuracy indicator depends on the possibility of determining, for a given task and set of materials, the range of error levels which are characteristic of normally efficient performance. In the present study these levels were determined by individual tests on the members of a sample of competent readers (see Chapter 5). A subject who produced error levels which lay outside these limits was then said to exhibit evidence of inefficiency in the processes or pathways involved in the performance of the task.

Error effects

The interpretative use of the accuracy index relies on demonstrations that particular psycholinguistic or processing factors exert a consistent influence on error levels. These accuracy effects were assessed by means of a chi-square test on the frequencies of correct and incorrect responses observed under the levels of the factor of interest. If the chi-square statistic exceeded the critical value for $p < 0.05$ then the effect on accuracy was said to be significant.

Classification of errors

In the investigations of acquired dyslexia it has been usual to assign error responses to various categories, e.g. semantic errors, visual errors, function word substitutions, derivational errors. This practice has its problems, most obviously that the errors, examined in a coded form subsequent to their production, may be ambiguous between categories. Nonetheless, it was considered worthwhile to attempt a simple classification of the error response produced in the present research. The following categories were used:

Lexicality (word versus non-word)
Error responses were classified as words or non-words. The frequencies of word and non-word responses to word and non-word targets were tabulated and tested for covariation of target and response lexicality or for a bias towards the production of words or non-words.

Semantic or derivational errors
An error was classified as 'derivational' if the target and response shared the same stem but differed in ending or inflection (e.g. singing → 'sings', hunger → 'hungry', beauty → 'beautiful'). Occasional errors which appeared to involve a semantic relationship (e.g. hotel → 'holiday') were included in this category.

Phonetic regularisation errors
An error was classified as a regularisation if the response was phonetically plausible on the basis of an application of grapheme-phoneme correspondence rules (e.g. canoe → 'canoh').

The remaining errors were described as 'translation errors'. These included all responses which appeared to be structurally related to their targets but to contain minor errors of letter identity or position. In practice, the great majority of errors fell into this category.

These error categories can be related to the information processing model. Error responses which are words are assumed often to be products of retrieval from the vocabulary store resulting from (1) a discrimination error in the morpheme recognition component of the visual processor, or (2) the referral of output from the grapheme-phoneme translator to the vocabulary store. Non-word errors, by contrast, are assumed to be products of grapheme-phoneme translation operation without lexical intervention. This is also true of phonetic regularisation errors. A semantic or derivational error, on the other hand, is thought to depend on an involvement of the semantic processor and its communication with the phonological processor.

Structural analysis of errors

A majority of the errors were classifiable as 'visual confusions' or 'translation failures'. An attempt was made to assess the degree of correspondence existing between the target and the response and also to determine which letter groups were most likely to be mis-translated. This was approached by representing error responses by a plausible orthography and by then parsing the target and the error into a series of vowel and consonant groups which were aligned and tested for correspondence. Where the error was a word its conventional spelling was used. If it was a non-word, correctly translated sounds were represented by the letters occurring in the target and errors by a conventional spelling.

The parsing of the arrays was carried out by a program which looked for vowels and vowel clusters (including combinations such as 'or', 'aw' and 'igh') and segregated each array into an alternating series of vowel and consonant clusters. If the arrays started with different categories or if they contained different numbers of clusters, the program attempted to find an alignment which maximised the correspondence. It then carried out a cluster by cluster comparison, scoring +1.0 for an exact match, +0.5 for a partial match, and 0.0 for a mismatch. The correspondence score was taken to be the total of the match scores expressed as a percentage of the number of clusters in the target. A distinction was made between vowel and consonant clusters and between simple clusters, containing only one letter and complex clusters containing more than one letter. To illustrate, the error: liberty → 'library' would be analysed as shown here in Table 4.2. This gives a correspondence score of 3.5 out of 6, which is 58 per cent. By carrying out this type of analysis on each error, it was possible to obtain an overall estimate of the degree of structural correspondence characterising an individual's error responses and also to determine whether mis-translations focused on vowels rather than on consonants, and on complex spelling patterns rather than on simple ones.

TABLE 4.2   *Analysis of error 'liberty' → 'library', into simple (S) or complex (C) vowel (V) and consonant (C) clusters*

Category	Target	Response	Score
SC	L	L	+1.0
SV	I	I	+1.0
SC	B	BR	+0.5
CV	ER	A	0.0
SC	T	R	0.0
SV	Y	Y	+1.0

4.8 Conclusions

This chapter has discussed practical considerations which arise when attempting to set up a procedure for the cognitive assessment of dyslexic problems. Given that an information processing model of basic reading functions is available, the requirement was seen as one of identifying a set of tasks and factor variations which could be mapped onto the model and then applied these to individual dyslexic and competent readers.

The methodology for doing this is divisible into three sub-parts: (1) procedures for designing and constructing experiments, (2) procedures for conduct of experiments, and (3) procedures for analysis and interpretation of data. In the present case, an effort was made to automate each of these sets of procedures on a microcomputer. At this level, the research depended on:

(1)   a set of programs for entry of vocabulary lists and construction of randomised and coded sequences;
(2)   programs for the display of stimuli in specified formats and the recording of reaction times and responses;
(3)   programs for summarising the experimental records and carrying out statistical tests of the significance of effects.

Once assembled, this procedure rendered the practical task of setting up and running experiments and summarising and analysing the data of individuals relatively straightforward.

5 Cognitive analysis of competent reading

5.1 Introduction

The objective of this research is to explore the hypothesis that dyslexic disorders derive from inefficiencies in particular components of the information processing system underlying reading competence. In order to approach this objective it is necessary to carry out an evaluative treatment of the dyslexic data and this depends on the availability of standards against which the efficiency of specified processes can be assessed.

A first requirement, therefore, is for information about the performance of normally competent readers on the experimental tasks. I did not have the resources to undertake an extensive normative investigation and decided to restrict myself to a study of a small sample of competent readers who were somewhat younger than my dyslexic cases. The dyslexic subjects were all adolescents or young adults of secondary school age and above. I considered that it would be permissible to take the data of competent readers at the upper primary level (i.e. aged about 11 years) as a definition of efficient performance which could be used to evaluate the results of older dyslexic subjects.

In Chapter 1, I noted that many studies of normal reading have been based on the presumption in favour of homogeneity and that it has been standard practice to report results in the form of group averages. There were at least two reasons why it seemed undesirable that this practice should be followed in the present instance. Since it was intended that the dyslexic data should be analysed at the level of individuals, it seemed essential that the results of the competent readers should be treated in the same way. It was also possible that the competent reader sample would prove to be heterogeneous, either on account of strategic differences between subjects or because of the presence of minor impairments in subjects who were competent on formal criteria.

5.2 General method

Two locally situated schools were approached and asked if they would agree to co-operate in the testing of some competent readers from the top primary class. A third school was asked to provide children who had difficulty in reading and who were considered to be in need of remedial tuition. A sample of 22 subjects was obtained in this way.

Each child was given an intellectual assessment, using an abbreviated version of the WISC-R. Reading and spelling were testing by the Schonell graded word lists. The children were classified as 'competent' if their reading age was at or in advance of their chronological age and as 'impaired' if the reading age was behind the chronological age.

Table 5.1 gives the details of the ages, IQ scores and reading and spelling assessments of the members of the sample who were classifiable as 'competent' according to the above criterion. The subjects are identified by their initials which will be used to refer to individuals during the presentation of the data. They were in general of above average verbal intelligence, although two of the children from the second school (PB and JD) showed a marked verbal-performance discrepancy. All subjects other than PM and JS were also in advance of their chronological ages on the spelling test.

TABLE 5.1   *Details of members of the sample of competent readers (Groups A and B).*

Group	School	Initials	Sex	Age	WISC–R Verbal IQ	Performance IQ	Schonell Reading age	Spelling age
	I	NT	m	12-3	144	146	12-6+	13-11
	I	JK	m	11-10	125	121	12-6+	12-6
A	I	PM	m	11-11	116	118	12-4	10-10
	I	AD	f	11-9	129	118	12-6+	12-0
	I	AL	m	11-7	131	114	12-3	12-2
	I	LH	f	11-10	125	118	12-3	12-11
	I	LM	f	12-0	110	111	12-6+	11-4
	II	PB	m	10-9	125	72	12-1	13-5
	II	JS	f	11-6	131	146	12-3	11-1
B	II	KH	m	11-11	135	107	12-6+	13-7
	II	JD	m	11-0	116	76	12-6+	12-4
	I	KB	f	12-0	106	90	12-6+	12-6
	II	LL	f	11-0	119	125	11-4	11-8

Each child completed a series of 11 experiments which formed the 'core' of the cognitive assessment procedure. These experiments were identified in Table 4.1. They may be subdivided along the lines of the earlier discussion to distinguish between:

(1)   tests of route 'm' to phonology (word vocalisation tasks);
(2)   tests of route 'g' to phonology (non-word reading tasks);
(3)   tests of route 'm' to semantics (lexical and semantic decision tasks);
(4)   tests on the visual processor (matching tasks, format distortions).

The experiments were all conducted by individual testing with the Apple II microcomputer. The children from the first school came to the Department of Psychology for testing. The others were tested in a quiet room which was made available in their school. The apparatus and procedure were as described in Chapter 4.

5.3 Vocalisation of words

The task of reading aloud words of varying familiarity was employed as a procedure for testing the performance characteristics of the morphemic route to phonology. These can be defined in terms of overall reaction time and accuracy levels and by reference to the effects of the relevant variables of frequency of usage, word length, spelling-to-sound regularity and abstract versus concrete meaning.

Distribution of vocal reaction times

As a first step, the reaction time distributions for correct responses to high and low frequency words were plotted for each subject. Inspection established that some subjects produced only responses in adjacent categories at the fast end of the scale whereas others made occasional very slow responses. These configurations correspond to the Type A and Type B reaction time distributions described in Chapter 4.

The subjects who produced well-formed distributions containing no slow or outlying responses were assigned to Group A. Subjects whose distributions included one or more outlying responses were placed in Group B. It was considered that this tendency to produce occasional slow responses when reading words might be indicative of a mild inefficiency affecting the operation of route 'm' to phonology. This 'morphemic effect' was noteworthy only in the cases of LL, KB and JS.

Frequency effect

A second way of assessing the efficiency of the morphemic channel is by considering the magnitude of the impact of variations in word frequency on performance. The relevant data have been summarised in Table 5.2. In

Group A, all subjects other than JK responded significantly faster to high frequency words than to low frequency words. The 'frequency effect' ranged from 39 ms for NT to 70 ms for AL. In Group B the only subject who did not show an effect was JD. This boy's results were distorted by one very slow response to a high frequency word. When the data were reanalysed with this outlier removed there was significant frequency effect of 35 ms. KB, JS and LL differed from the remainder of the sample in showing an exaggerated frequency effect (see Table 5.2).

TABLE 5.2   *Range of values for (1) mean reaction time (ms), (2) standard deviation of the reaction time distribution (ms), (3) slope of linear function relating reaction time to word length (ms/letter), and (4) error rates (per cent) for the competent readers*

	High frequency words	Low frequency words	Frequency effect
RT range	577-752	616-816	35-93
sd range	70-207	74-318	
Slope	0-23	6-33	
Error	0-3	2-10	
JS			
RT	657	831	174
sd	113	459	
Slope	−2	13	
Error	0	7.14	
KB			
RT	791	977	186
sd	360	612	
Slope	31	35	
Error	0	2.04	
LL			
RT	1028	1167	139
sd	428	583	
Slope	48	24	
Error	0.72	6.12	

If the results of these three subjects are left aside, the characteristics of normally efficient performance for reading high and low frequency words might be summarised in the following terms:

High frequency words
The mean reaction time should fall within the range 570-760 ms with a standard deviation between 70-210 ms and errors on fewer than 4 per cent of trials.

Low frequency words

The mean reaction time should fall between 610 ms and 820 ms with a standard deviation 70-320 ms and between 2 and 10 per cent of errors. The mean reaction time for low frequency words is likely to exceed the mean for high frequency words by 30-100 ms.

Inclusion of the data of JS, KB and LL would raise the time estimates to about 1000 ms (sd = 400 ms) for high frequency words and to 1200 ms (sd = 600 ms) for low frequency words, with a frequency effect of up to 200 ms.

Length effects

The high and low frequency words presented to the subjects in Experiments 1 and 2 varied in length between 3 and 7 letters. If the visual analysis underlying the operation of route 'm' to phonology involves a serial process, then it would be expected that the reaction time should increase as a linear function of the number of letters in the word. If, on the other hand, recognition can be achieved by an approximation to a parallel process, then there need be no consistent relationship between word length and reaction time. In order to assess this effect the slope and intercept parameters of the lines of best fit to the relation between reaction time and word length were calculated.

Leaving aside the results of KB and LL, the slope values obtained for high frequency words fell within a range of −2 ms/letter to 23 ms/letter. In general, a significant linear trend was detectable with slope values of 16 ms/letter or greater. KB and LL, analysed with outliers >2500 ms removed, gave values of 31 ms/letter and 48 ms/letter.

These data do not give an unequivocal answer to the question of whether route 'm' to phonology typically operates as a serial or a parallel process. They do, however, indicate that the processing rate is very fast (25 ms/letter or less) and statistically negligible in a proportion of subjects.

5.4 Non-word reading

According to the theoretical assumptions set out earlier, the operation of route 'g' to phonology can be assessed by taking performance measures in the task of reading aloud non-words. A summary of the results obtained from the competent readers on this task appears in Table 5.3.

The difference between word and non-word reading, to be referred to as the 'lexicality effect', was defined as the reaction time and accuracy difference between non-words and low frequency words. The non-word

TABLE 5.3   *Vocal reaction times (ms), standard deviations (ms), slope of function relating reaction time to non-word length (ms/letter), and error rates (per cent) for non-word reading by the competent readers*

Subject	Vocal reaction time (ms)	Standard deviation (ms)	Slope (ms/letter)	Error rate (%)
Group A	787-1002	195-466	28-42	1-16
JK	821	148	15	24.17
Group B				
JD	973	343	37	5.83
LM	1176	512	48	15.00
PB	1286	1008	107	8.33
KH	1303	533	33	5.00
KB	1214	423	74	8.33
JS	2411	2433	396	15.13
LL	2122	1103	148	5.00

distributions tended to be more widely dispersed than low frequency word distributions (KB is the only exception), and to have a higher mean. In Group A, the lexicality effect ranged from 119 ms to 212 ms. In Group B, JD's results appear similar to the Group A data, but the other subjects all showed some evidence of an exaggeration of the lexicality effect, attributable mainly to the appearance of outlying responses in the distributions. The effect was moderate in the cases of LM, PB and KH but quite substantial for JS and LL, both of whom had mean reaction times above 2000 ms and distributions which contained numerous slow responses. This exaggeration of the lexicality effect will be referred to as a 'phonological effect' localised in route 'g' and can be distinguished from the 'morphemic effect' mentioned in the preceding section.

Considering only the subjects who showed no evident phonological effects (the Group A subjects plus JD), the characteristics of efficient non-word reading might be summarised as follows:

Efficient non-word reading
The mean reaction time should fall between 780 ms and 1000 ms with a standard deviation of 140-470 ms and between 1 and 16 per cent errors. The reaction time difference between non-words and low frequency words should fall within the range 110-220 ms.

In estimating the upper bound for the error rate at about 16 per cent I have disregarded the results of the Group A subject, JK. This boy had very fast reaction time levels and very compact distributions but made over 24 per cent of errors in non-word reading. This error rate was well clear of all other subjects in the sample and I have accordingly taken it to be indicative of an unusual degree of imprecision in the translation process. JK's results indicate that a phonological effect on accuracy may occur in the absence of an effect on reaction time, and that inaccuracy in non-word reading is compatible with very accurate reading of words. This suggests that the operation of route 'm' to phonology is not compromised when route 'g' becomes liable to error.

The results of LM, PB, KH and JS carry similar implications. These subjects all showed a delay in reading non-words which did not extend to their reading of words. A functional differentiation between routes 'g' and 'm' is implied. I will take the results of the first three subjects to be representative of performance levels associated with a 'mild phonological effect'. These levels can be estimated in the following terms:

Mild phonological effect
Non-words are read with a mean reaction time between 1100 ms and
1300 ms and a standard deviation of 500-1000 ms. The difference
between non-words and low frequency words fall in the range 480-570 ms.

The data of subject JS showed a more extreme effect which appears relatively severe within the context of this sample of readers. She had a reaction time of over 2400 ms and a lexicality effect of nearly 1600 ms. Figure 5.1 gives a plot of JS's word and non-word reaction time distributions. These results are strikingly similar to those of dyslexic subjects who show a large phonological impairment combined with relatively efficient morphemic processing.

If the results of LL are taken as an indication of the lower bound for the identification of these more severe effects, then the following definition of impaired functioning within route 'g' to phonology could be proposed:

Marked phonological effect
The reaction time in non-word reading exceeds 2000 ms with a standard
deviation greater than 1000 ms and a distribution which contains a
substantial tail of very slow responses extending to 4000 ms and beyond.
The lexicality effect may be 1000 ms or more.

If a non-word reading involves a process of grapheme-phoneme translation in which familiar letter clusters are identified and used to retrieve their phonemic equivalents, and if this segmenting process operates in a serial fashion, then the reaction to vocalise non-words will be expected to increase as a function of non-word length. Table 5.3 includes the slope values obtained by fitting straight lines to the non-word reading data of each subject. The linear trend test was significant for all subjects other than JK in Group A and KH in Group B. Following removal

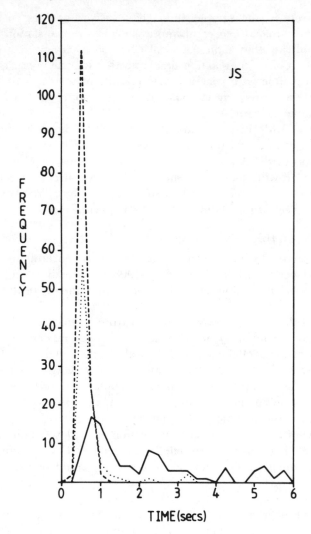

FIGURE 5.1   *Plot of reaction time distributions for correct responses to high frequency words*
(– – –), low frequency (. . .) words and non-words (——) by the competent reader JS

of outliers, the slope values for the phonologically efficient subjects were
found to lie within a range of 28 ms/letter to 42 ms/letter. The analysis of
the mildly affected subjects gave values between 48 ms/letter and
107 ms/letter. The rates for the strongly affected subjects, LL and JS, were
148 ms/letter and 396 ms/letter.

These results support the conclusion that, in competent readers, a fast
serial process is often involved in grapheme-phoneme translation. This
differential effect of length on word and non-word reading may help to

explain why the distributions of reaction times for non-words tend to have a higher mean and somewhat wider dispersion than the distributions for words.

5.5 Psycholinguistic effects

The vocabularies used in the word reading experiments varied on dimensions of form class and abstract versus concrete meaning in one study and on a dimension of spelling-to-sound regularity in another. The non-word vocabulary incorporated a variation in the homophony of the items. These factors were introduced with the objective of detecting concurrent supportive processing during the operation of routes 'm' and 'g' to phonology.

The possible effects on word reading will be considered first. If semantic processing plays a significant role in the retrieval of responses to words, and if abstract semantics constitute a less effective basis for retrieval than concrete semantics, then it is to be expected that function words will be read less efficiently than content words, and that abstract words will be read less efficiently than concrete words. If, on the other hand, response retrieval is supported by grapheme-phoneme translation, and if irregular words create conflicts between the output of the translator and the response retrieved from the vocabulary store, then reading will show reductions in efficiency for irregular words.

According to standard models of dyslexic disorders (Marshall and Newcombe, 1973; Shallice, 1981), a morphemic dyslexia is expected to increase reliance on grapheme-phoneme translation and hence to exaggerate effects of spelling irregularity. A phonological dyslexia, on the other hand, should reduce the involvement of the translation process, and a consequence of this should be that regularity effect will be less evident in subjects having a phonological impairment than in subjects having an unimpaired translator. It is also possible that an impairment of route 'g' will lead to an increased reliance on semantic processing, resulting in an exaggeration of the effects of form class and abstract meaning. If these generalisations are applicable for competent readers who give evidence of mild morphemic or phonological effects, then phonological subjects, such as LM, PB, KH and JS, should give reduced evidence of regularity effects and enhanced evidence of syntactic/semantic effects. Subjects such as KB and LL, who displayed a mild morphemic effect, might be expected to show the opposite pattern, although it must be remembered that LL presented a combined morphemic and phonological effect.

Comparisons were made, for each subject individually, between function words and high frequency content words and between concrete and abstract words at each level of frequency, using a t-test to compare reaction

TABLE 5.4 *Mean vocal reaction times (ms) and error rates for reading regular and irregular words, and homophonic and non-homophonic non-words*

Group	Subject		High frequency words		Low frequency words		Non-words	
			Regular	Irregular	Regular	Irregular	Homophones	Non-homophones
	NT	X̄	601	593	595	655[1]	790	785
		sd	100	45	45	91	220	165
		E%	0	0	0	7.14	0	1.67
	JK	X̄	589	593	607	627	799	845
		sd	48	68	78	82	128	165
		E%	0	3.57	0	17.86[2]	20	28.33
	PM	X̄	651	664	658	737[1]	797	863[3]
		sd	173	121	79	143	192	174
		E%	3.57	0	3.57	14.29	11.67	20
A	AD	X̄	699	582	701	848[1]	925	987
		sd	109	69	79	214	589	276
		E%	0	0	3.57	7.14	1.67	8.33
	AL	X̄	631	654	694	754[1]	924	991
		sd	100	76	101	127	277	264
		E%	0	0	0	7.14	3.33	10
	LH	X̄	666	669	702	811[1]	973	1038
		sd	92	147	153	160	244	272
		E%	0	3.57	3.57	17.86	3.33	20[4]

TABLE 5.4 *Continued*

LM	X̄	642	612	641	820[1]	1098	1258
	sd	151	78	86	224	432	573
	E%	0	7.14	3.57	7.14	13.33	16.67
PB	X̄	622	638	655	882[1]	1074	1514[3]
	sd	85	162	117	535	379	1362
	E%	3.57	3.57	3.57	7.14	5	11.67
JS	X̄	679	694	744	997[1]	1930	2962[3]
	sd	109	114	161	565	1469	3111
	E%	0	0	0	21.43[2]	10	20.34
B KH	X̄	714	776	722	802[1]	1137	1475[3]
	sd	153	402	95	193	439	567
	E%	0	0	0	10.71	3.33	6.67
JD	X̄	705	738	753	802	901	1041[3]
	sd	71	116	159	182	156	443
	E%	0	3.57	0	21.43[2]	8.33	3.33
KB	X̄	772	666	809	1014	1114	1322[3]
	sd	554	66	405	777	393	427
	E%	0	0	0	3.57	5	11.67
LL	X̄	915	1058	1067	1100	1762	2496[3]
	sd	317	564	461	465	853	1203
	E%	0	0	0	17.86[2]	3.33	6.67

[1] Regularity effect on low frequency words at p<0.05 or better by t-test.
[2] Regularity effect on accuracy at p<0.05 or better by χ^2 test.
[3] Homophony effect on non-word reading at p<0.05 or better by t-test
[4] Homophony effect on accuracy at p<0.05 or better by χ^2 test.

time distributions and a chi-square test to compare error frequencies. Where appropriate, the reaction time data were analysed with extreme outliers removed.

The Group A subjects were in general not affected by the form class variable, the one exception being AD who showed a significant delay when responding to function words. There was also little evidence of effects of abstract meaning. The exceptions were AD's reading of high frequency words and LH's reading of low frequency words. In Group B the subjects who were expected to show semantic effects were LM, PB, KH and JS. There was some support for this in the results of PB and JS, but not for LM or KH.

These results are obviously far from clear-cut and suggest that the incidence of semantic effects within a sample of competent readers may be somewhat variable and not unequivocally related to the presence or absence of a phonological inefficiency. It is also true that those effects which were observed tended to influence high frequency word reading, whereas the more natural expectation is that semantic processing should contribute to the slower process of low frequency word retrieval.

The effects of the spelling-to-sound regularity variable have been summarised in Table 5.4. Individual comparisons were made between regular and irregular words at each level of frequency. With the exception of JK, all of the Group A subjects showed significant effects of irregularity on the speed of reading low frequency words. The regularity effect varied between 60 ms and 147 ms. In JK's case, there was a significant effect on accuracy of reading low frequency words. An accuracy effect was also shown by subject JD in Group B.

The theoretical expectation that the Group B subjects who gave evidence of a phonological inefficiency should not show a regularity effect was clearly not supported by the data. JS, the subject exhibiting the strongest phonological effect, read low frequency irregular words significantly more slowly and less accurately than the low frequency regular words. Likewise, LM, PB and KH all showed significant reaction time effects, ranging from 80 ms to 179 ms. Some regularity effects also appeared in the data of KB and LL.

Half of the items in the non-word list were homophones of English words. If non-words are read via an independent grapheme-phoneme translator, then homophony should not influence performance unless the output from the channel is lexicalised by being matched against entries in the vocabulary store. The effects of this variable have been summarised in Table 5.4. The Group A subjects were relatively unaffected by homophony, the exceptions being a reaction time effect by PM and an accuracy effect by LH. Much clearer effects occurred in Group B. All subjects other than LM responded faster to homophonic non-words than to the non-homophones. Leaving aside subjects JS and LL, the effect ranged from 140 ms to 440 ms.

The effects for JS and LL were 1032 ms and 734 ms respectively. These results suggest that the most efficient readers in the sample read non-words without reference to the speech production lexicon. Readers who gave evidence of phonological inefficiency tended to seek lexical support for the translation process.

The non-word vocabulary also included a variation in the complexity of the vowel structure. No Group A subject showed any effect of this variable. However, in Group B subjects LM, PB, JS and KB all made more errors on complex vowels than on simple vowels.

5.6 Error classification

The error responses produced by the subjects in the word and non-word vocalisation experiments were assembled and submitted to two types of analysis: (1) a classification of error types, and (2) a structural analysis designed to quantify the similarity of error responses and their targets and to assess the relative contributions of vowel and consonant clusters to the errors.

The 'lexicality' of error responses was considered first. If most errors were generated by the speech production lexicon, then it would be expected that a majority would be words. If, on the other hand, errors were generated by a grapheme-phoneme translator operating without reference to the morphemic systems, then a substantial proportion of errors should be non-words (neologisms). Table 5.5 gives the frequencies of word and non-word error responses to word and non-word targets. It seems clear that all subjects produced a mixture of word and non-word responses and that response lexicality was not directly determined by target lexicality. The occurrence of a reasonable number of neologisms implies that a proportion of errors were generated by the translation channel.

The table also shows the latencies of the error responses. If errors were often generated by the grapheme-phoneme translator, then it should follow that subjects exhibiting an impairment of this sub-system should also have high error reaction times. The results of LL and JS show precisely this expected elevation of the error latency. The case of JS is particularly instructive. Her error responses were made very slowly and a substantial proportion of them were non-word responses to non-words. This is consistent with the earlier conclusion that, despite her phonological impairment, she made extensive use of the translation channel when reading.

The errors were also examined with a view to classifying the relationship existing between the target and the response. A majority of errors were most obviously classifiable as 'translation failures', involving confusions over letter identities, positions or order, or 'visual confusions' between

TABLE 5.5   *Reaction times (ms) and frequencies of word and non-word error responses to word and non-word targets by the competent readers*

| | | Word target | | Non-word target | |
		Word	Non-word	Word	Non-word
RT range		655-1046	652-1807	958-1639	1109-2688
	N.	1-5	1-8	6-19	2-19
JK	RT	734	751	854	1027
	N.	7	4	15	32
JS	RT	2057	2515	3785	3720
	N.	4	6	11	25
LL	RT	2211	1911	2888	3550
	N.	2	6	4	6

words (e.g. liberty → 'library'). There were no instances of errors involving a semantic or derivational relationship between the target and the response. However, most subjects produced occasional errors which were classifiable as 'phonetic regularisations' (e.g. come → 'comb').

A further analysis involved an assessment of the structural relationship between the target and the response. This was based on the parsing and matching procedure which was described in Chapter 4. A summary of the outcome of this analysis appears in Table 5.6. Two points emerge quite clearly. The first is that the major source of translation errors is to be found in the complex clusters, especially the vowels. For example, subject JK, who made a large number of errors in non-word reading, made 21 per cent of correct translations for complex vowels, 55 per cent for complex consonants, 65 per cent for simple vowels and 83 per cent for simple consonants. A similar pattern appears in the data of several other subjects. A second point is that error responses were generally structurally close to their targets. The table provides two indices of structural similarity. One is the percentage of items in each subject's error set having a similarity score below 50 per cent. This ranges from 0 per cent for subject KB to 25 per cent for subject AL. Another is the average value of the similarity scores computed for each of the errors. These averages fell between 64 per cent and 76 per cent. A third possible index is the percentage match score obtained by summing the scores for the complete sample of clusters included in the subject's error set. This figure ranged from 63 per cent to 82 per cent.

TABLE 5.6   *Ranges of percentage match scores for simple and complex vowels and consonants, per cent of errors with match scores below 50 per cent, and average similarity of errors and targets for the competent readers*

Group	Simple Consonants	Vowels	Complex Consonants	Vowels	Match <50%	Average similarity
A	62-83	52-65	51-66	0-25	5-23	64-70
B	64-94	41-92	33-76	12-50	0-20	64-75

5.7 Lexical and semantic decision tasks

The semantic decision task was employed as a procedure for assessing the functioning of route 'm' to semantics. Subjects were presented with names of categories followed by names of instances which they classified as category members or non-members by a Yes or No response. The typicality of positive instances and the relatedness of the negatives were varied.

Table 5.7 contains a summary of the semantic decision results. For Group A, the mean reaction time fell within the range 800-1450 ms with a standard deviation of 250-650 ms and 10-20 per cent of errors. If an impairment of route 'm' to phonology is likely to be accompanied by a parallel effect on route 'm' to semantics, it would be expected that the Group B subjects KB and LL should show delays in the semantic decision task. This appears not to have happened for KB, although LL does have an elevated reaction time level, which, at over 2000 ms, lies well outside the range for the remaining subjects.

Typicality and relatedness effects were somewhat variably distributed. Typicality affected reaction time or accuracy for seven of the subjects and all, other than LL, showed some relatedness effects. An error rate of about 10 per cent seems to be typical, with the higher rates shown by AD, LH and LM being mainly attributable to mistakes on the related negative items.

It was anticipated that semantic decisions would be likely to involve a parallel visual analysis process. However, the slopes of the word length functions which have been included in Table 5.7 were all positive and the tests of linear trend were significant for all subjects other than NT, PM, KH and LL. The significant slope values ranged from 38 ms/letter to 142 ms/letter.

On the basis of these data the characteristics of normally efficient performance in the semantic decision task might be summarised in the following terms:

Semantic decisions

The mean reaction time should fall between 830 ms and 1590 ms with a standard deviation of 250-640 ms and about 8-12 per cent of errors. Processing may appear serial with a rate of up to 150 ms/letter.

This definition treats the error rates of 15-20 per cent shown by three of the subjects as indicative of a possible inefficiency. A reaction time of 2000 ms or more is treated as evidence of a possible morphemic inefficiency, especially when the distribution contains a tail of slow responses.

Table 5.7 presents a summary of the results from the lexical decision task in which subjects discriminated between words of high and low frequency and legal or illegal non-words. In Group A, reaction times fell within the range 660 ms to 1060 ms with a standard deviation of 145 ms to 315 ms and between 7 and 13 per cent of errors. The range for Group B was from 660 ms to 1160 ms, with subject LL's reaction time of over 1400 ms again lying outside the main distribution.

TABLE 5.7   *Mean reaction times (ms), standard deviations (ms), slopes of functions relating reaction time to word length (ms/letter), and error rates (per cent) for semantic and lexical decisions by the competent readers*

	Semantic decisions	Lexical decisions
RT range	832-1585	660-1076
sd range	253-635	153-391
Slope (ms/letter)	21-142	−7-31
Error (%)	8-20	5-14
KB		
RT	1261	1154
sd	369	189
Slope	70	20
Error	5.83	8.33
LL		
RT	2091	1454
sd	827	711
Slope	66	46
Error	9.17	9.17

The subjects all showed effects of legality on negative reaction time or accuracy. Illegal non-words were rejected virtually without error with a reaction time between 800 ms and 1360 ms. All subjects other than LH, LM and JS showed effects of word frequency on the reaction time or accuracy of positive responses.

Inspection of the error patterns suggests the presence of strategic differences. The subjects were all good at discriminating high frequency words and illegal non-words. Some also achieved good discrimination between low frequency words and legal non-words (PM, LH, PB, JS, KH, JD and LL). The overall error rate for these subjects fell within a range of 5 per cent to 10 per cent. The remaining subjects were characterised by high error levels on the legal non-words, reaching 50 per cent for JK, AL and AD, and 75 per cent for LM. It seems that these subjects adopted a strategy of responding positively to items having a legal orthographic structure. Subject KB was atypical in that she had a high error rate (over 40 per cent) on low frequency words combined with fully accurate performance on legal non-words. It seems likely that her strategy was to respond negatively to all items which were not immediately recognisable as familiar words.

The existence of these strategic variations makes it difficult to estimate the characteristics of efficient performance on the lexical decision task. A statement based on the data of the subjects achieving good discrimination might be:

Lexical decisions
The mean reaction time should fall within the range 660 ms to 1080 ms with a standard deviation between 150 ms and 400 ms and between 5 and 10 per cent of errors.

This definition treats error rates above about 30 per cent on either legal non-words or low frequency words as indicative of poor discrimination, attributable either to a strategic curtailment of search and checking processes or to a true morphemic impairment. Given that competent readers appear willing to tolerate quite high rates of error on this task, it may be preferable to rely on the reaction time as an indicator of morphemic impairment. Thus, subject LL, while achieving good discrimination, has an elevated mean reaction time and a dispersed distribution which includes a tail of slow responses.

Table 5.7 also contains the slope values of lines fitted to the lexical decision data. In contrast to the semantic decision results, there were no instances of significant linear trends of reaction time against word length. This was also true of responses to illegal non-words for all subjects other than JD. The slopes for responses to legal non-words were generally positive and were quite large in some instances. Linear trends were significant for JS, KH and JD with rates between 60 and 75 ms/letter.

5.8 Visual matching tasks

Two experimental procedures were applied with the aim of assessing the visual processor component of the model: (1) the identity matching task, and (2) the array matching task. A summary of the results from both experiments appears in Table 5.8.

TABLE 5.8   *Summary of reaction time (ms) and error data for identity matching and array matching by the competent readers. Slope values give the relation between reaction time and display size for identity matching, and the position of difference function for array matching*

Group			Identity matching	Array matching
A		RT	699-778	1056-1454
		sd	131-221	297-518
		slope	−8-10	22-160
		Error %	1-6	2-17
	LH	RT	1730	2262
		sd	881	911
		slope	6	221
		Error %	5	6
B		RT	801-1328	1242-1843
		sd	197-567	349-572
		slope	−8-16	16-245
		Error %	1-8	5-18
	LL	RT	1353	2315
		sd	580	923
		slope	21	445
		Error %	3.62	10

The mean reaction time of the Group A subjects on the identity matching task fell between 690 ms and 780 ms, with fewer than 6 per cent of errors. Subject LH stood out as distinct from the others with a mean of over 1700 ms and the dispersed distribution. Reaction times were somewhat higher in Group B and errors fell in the range 1-8 per cent. LL and PB had relatively high means and dispersed distributions. If these are considered to be atypical, the range for Group B lies between 730 ms and 1280 ms with a standard deviation of 190-360 ms.

The involvement of parallel processing in identity matching tasks is best considered on the basis of estimates of the effects of display size on the Yes reaction time. In Group A the obtained slope values were either negative or negligibly small and there were no instances of significant linear trends. This was also generally true of the Group B subjects, although KB and JS had significant processing rates of 18 ms/letter and 29 ms/letter.

A definition of efficient performance in the identity matching experiment might then be formulated in the following terms:

Identity matching
The mean reaction time should fall within the range 690 ms to 1300 ms

with a standard deviation of 130 ms to 360 ms and between 0 and 8 per cent of errors. Positive reaction time should not increase as a function of the number of letters presented for matching.

On this criterion, subjects LH, PB and LL could be said to have reaction time levels which are high enough to suggest the presence of a mild visual processor inefficiency.

The results of the array matching experiment have been included in Table 5.8. In Group A, the mean reaction time fell within a range of 1050 ms to 1460 ms with a standard deviation between 290 ms and 520 ms and 2-17 per cent of errors. Subject LH again stood out from the others by her high mean and dispersed distribution. In Group B the main set of reaction times lay between 1100 ms and 1850 ms. Subject LL was differentiated from the others by the mean level and degree of dispersion of her distribution.

All subjects other than PM, PB, KH and KB showed significant effects on positive reaction time of the variation in orthographic legality. There were also occasional effects on accuracy or negative reaction time. These 'legality effects' confirm the results of numerous previous investigations and are interpreted as evidence for the availability of a model of English orthography which has been internalised within the visual processor.

In order to examine properties of the processing involved in array comparisons, a 'position of difference' function was calculated for the negative trials on which the letter sets differed at one position only. The slope values of this function have been included in Table 5.8. A large value of the index associated with a significant linear trend is suggestive of a serial self-terminating procedure, operating from left to right across the display. Only subjects AL and LH in Group A gave evidence of directed processing of this kind. In Group B, all subjects other than KH and KB had significant slope values, ranging from 133 ms/position for JS to 245 ms/position for PB. Subject LL's processing rate was very slow at 445 ms/position. These results suggest that the adoption of a serial left-to-right scan is a strategic option which is taken up by some subjects but not by others. It seems that LL's high mean reaction time in matching was at least partly attributable to her use of a very slow serial procedure in making the comparisons.

The following can be proposed as a definition of efficient performance in the array matching task:

Array matching
The mean reaction time should fall within a range of 1050-1850 ms with a standard deviation of 290-580 ms and an error rate of 2-18 per cent.
Legal arrays should be matched faster than illegal arrays.

According to this criterion, subject LH in Group A and subject LL in Group B gave evidence to an impairment of analytic visual processor functions. This confirms the indications provided by the identity matching data. In LL's case, slowness of visual matching was accompanied by delays in the other decision tasks as well as in the vocalisation tasks. This was not the case for LH, who presents a coincidence of efficient central processing and impaired visual processor functions. Hence, the processing delays shown by LL cannot be attributed to a visual processor defect since it is evident from the results of LH that such a defect does not necessarily compromise the central reading functions.

5.9 Format distortion effects

The second main approach to the analysis of visual processor functions involved the imposition of a load on the processor within the context of the vocalisation and decision tasks used to assess the central reading functions. In these experiments the word and non-word targets were presented in a standard horizontal format or with a zigzag or vertical rearrangement of the letter positions. The format distortion variation was combined with a variation in word length. The intention was to determine whether distortion impaired accuracy or reaction time, and, if so, whether the effect took the form of an increase in processing time per letter.

Table 5.9 gives summaries of the effects of distortions on the tasks of (1) reading words aloud, (2) reading non-words aloud, (3) making semantic decisions, and (4) making lexical decisions. The table gives the slopes of the lines of best fit to the relationship between reaction time and word length.

The data for the word vocalisation task will be considered first. There were no effects of distortion on reading accuracy, although every subject showed a significant reaction time effect, generally larger for the vertical than for the zigzag distortions. Although the zigzag distortion appeared to be associated with a slowing of processing rate, the linear trend tests were significant only in the cases of LH in Group A and JS, KB and LL in Group B. The vertical distortion, by contrast, was associated with slow serial processing with a rate between 50 ms/letter and 260 ms/letter in all subjects.

The non-word reading results are complicated by the presence, in Group B, of some subjects with phonological impairments. The Group A data reveal a variety of patterns. Distortion was associated with a significant rise in error rate for PM, NT, AD and AL. Evidence of serial reading can be found in the results of PN, AD, AL and LH. Subject JK, on the other hand, read the distorted non-words rapidly though inaccurately

TABLE 5.9   *Slope values (ms/letter) for reading of normal, zigzag and vertical formats in the vocalisation and decision tasks by the competent readers*

Format	Vocalisation		Decision	
	Words	Non-words	Semantic	Lexical
Normal	−30/33	−38/463	−54/123	−28/33
Zigzag	15/149	96/493	4/81	12/282
Vertical	49/257	−1/528	−15/208	15/393
LH				
Normal	−30	61	−18	28
Zigzag	65	213	47	55
Vertical	64	271	−2	224
LL				
Normal	45	142	17	2
Zigzag	337	160	−20	153
Vertical	244	681	9	358

and without resort to serial processing. NT also sustained fast processing rates although at the expense of some loss in accuracy. In Group B serial processing was apparent in the results of LM, KH, JB and KB. The rates were between 90 and 190 ms/letter for the zigzag displays and between 110 and 320/ms/letter for the vertical distortion. Subjects PB, JS and LL had processing rates which lay outside this range, approximating 500 ms/letter for PB and JS and well over 600 ms/letter for LL's reading of vertical non-words.

In the semantic decision experiment the processing rates were generally somewhat faster than in the vocalisation tasks. Most subjects gave evidence of serial processing when dealing with the vertical words but the rates were generally no slower than 200 ms/letter. Subjects who read the distorted items without resort to serial processing were PM and LH in Group A (though with an error cost for PM) and LL in Group B.

The lexical decision task also provided evidence that some subjects were able to process the distortions without resort to serial processing (e.g. NT and PM in Group A). Among the remainder, the rates for vertical words lay between 80 and 180 ms/letter, except for PB and LL, whose rates approximated 350-400 ms/letter.

A general specification of the effects of format distortion can be proposed on the basis of these data:

Format distortion effects
Zigzag and vertical distortions increase reaction time while leaving error rates unaffected and are often resolved by a serial process functioning at a rate of less than 250 ms/letter.

This definition is subject to the qualification that error costs sometimes occur when non-words are read and that processing rates for non-words may be somewhat slower than for words.

One question to be considered is whether the matching tasks and the distortions tap the same aspects of visual processor functions. The subjects who were identified as having a possible visual processor impairment on the basis of the matching tasks were LH and LL. LH did not show unusually large distortion effects although in three instances her processing rates were in excess of 200 ms/letter. LL, on the other hand, had slow rates in word and non-word reading and lexical decisions. Another subject who stands out on account of slow processing times per letter is JS in the non-word reading tasks. This is probably a reflection of her tendency to process non-words by a slow serial process in any case, and does not reflect a special impact of the distortions.

It seems reasonable to suggest that processing rates of up to about 200-250 ms/letter lie within a normal range, but that rates of 300 ms/letter and above could be regarded as indicative of a disturbance of the visual processor functions involved in resolving distortions.

5.10 Conclusions

This chapter has presented the results of an application of the cognitive assessment procedure to the members of a small sample of 11-year-old children who were competent readers according to standard criteria. The principal objective was to obtain estimates of the range of values for the reaction time and accuracy indicators which could be taken as represent-ative of efficient performance on the vocalisation and decision tasks. The experiments also provided information about the magnitudes of the effects of the factors which were varied. In what follows these estimates will be used as an approximate baseline to assist in the identification of efficient and impaired systems in dyslexic readers.

The study also permits some comments on the possibility that competent readers may show individual differences in strategy or efficiency.

Normally efficient reading

The first objective was to define normally efficient reading within the framework of the model. This is not a straightforward matter since the approach adopted depends on the manner in which some fundamental questions about the unit of analysis in cognitive research are addressed. In Chapter 2 I debated whether the reference of the term 'dyslexia' should be to processing configurations or to particular systems or sub-systems. My conclusion was that a preferred approach was one which emphasised the reference to systems and sub-systems rather than overall configurations. I think the same conclusion follows in the case of competent reading and that the right course is to start by definining the characteristics of efficient processing within each of the major routes postulated in the model without thereby accepting a commitment to the existence of a processing configuration which is considered to be standard among competent readers (i.e. a 'good reader' sub-type).

The model identifies four major domains within which normally efficient functioning may be defined. These are: (1) visual processor functions, (2) the morphemic route to phonology, (3) the grapheme-phoneme translation route to phonology,, and (4) the morphemic route to semantics. In the experimental analysis, efficiency of visual processor functions has been defined by reference to reaction time distributions and error levels in the visual matching tasks, the magnitude of the effects of word and non-word length on reaction time in the vocalisation and decision tasks, and the time or accuracy costs associated with format distortion resolution. Morphemically based access to phonology has been assessed by examining reaction time distributions and error levels in the task of reading aloud words of varying familiarity. Part of the definition of efficiency has been the requirement that the reaction time distribution should be well-formed, which has been taken to mean that the times should be grouped in a small number of adjacent categories at the fast end of the reaction time scale (Type A distribution). Similarly, the operation of the grapheme-phoneme translation route was defined in terms of accuracy levels and reaction time distributions in non-word reading, and the morphemic route to semantics by a consideration of the same indicators in the lexical and semantic decision tasks.

Strategic variations

The information processing model may be viewed as a specification of a set of options defined in terms of the pathways or combinations of pathways which are active during the performance of a particular task. The technique of identifying strategic differences in the choice among these options was to introduce into the experiments factor variations which were considered to have a localised reference. If a particular factor was found to exert a significant effect on reaction time or accuracy, then it should be possible to concude that a subject showing the effect was using the process influenced by the factor. If the effect was present for some subjects but not for others, then it could be concluded that the process in question was a strategic option which was taken up by some subjects but not by others. Similar arguments can be put forward in relation to the classification of errors. The

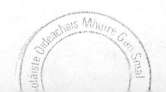

varieties of errors which were identified can be viewed as the products of distinct processing options. Hence, subjects producing errors of a given type may be assumed to be using the process of which the error type is characteristic. If the error types are produced by some subjects but not by others, then this again constitutes evidence for strategic variations among subjects.

A further area of optionality relates to the possibility of speed versus accuracy trading. A subject may make use of a particular process but may elect to maintain fast processing at the cost of quite high rates of error. Again, if this occurs for some subjects but not for others, then the presence of an element of optionality is indicated.

There were a number of aspects of the data which appeared helpful in identifying strategic variations between subjects. In the vocalisation experiments reading words with the support of concurrent processing through the semantic system was indexed by effects of form class and of abstract versus concrete meaning. This option was adopted only infrequently. Support by grapheme-phoneme translation was indexed by effects of spelling-to-sound irregularity and by the occurrence of phonetically regularised errors. This option was taken by a majority of subjects. In nonword reading, lexicalisation of the output from route 'g' was considered to be indexed by homophony effects. Again, this option was taken by some subjects but not by others.

The decision tasks gave further evidence of variations in the use of processing options. Some subjects matched letter arrays by a serial procedure which progressed systematically from left to right but others did not. The subjects also varied widely in their readiness to trade speed for accuracy in the lexical and semantic decision tasks, and in the extent to which they were affected by the typicality and relatedness variations.

Variations in efficiency

Aside from these strategic variations it seems clear that a sample of competent readers may be expected to include some subjects in whom all processing systems operate efficiently and others who give evidence of minor inefficiencies affecting one or more systems. These inefficiencies can also be defined by reference to the four major processing domains.

Morphemic effects
Inefficiency in word recognition and retrieval (route 'm' to phonology or route 'm' to semantics) is indexed by errors and slow responses when vocalising words or making lexical or semantic decisions or by exaggeration of the word frequency effect.

Phonological effect

An effect on route 'g' to phonology is marked by the occurrence of high rates of error or delayed reactions in the non-word reading task. These phonological effects do not necessary compromise the operation of the morphemic routes.

Visual processor effects

Inefficiency of visual processor functions is indexed by slow responses in the matching tasks, serial reading or slowness in resolving format distortions. These effects appeared not to have any necessary implications for the efficiency of the central functions.

Conclusion

This preliminary study of competent reading provides a necessary background to the investigation of dyslexic reading which is the main purpose of this monograph. The normal data provide quantitative definitions of efficient processing within each of the systems and pathways postulated in the model and also indicate which processes are subject to strategic variations and which ones can give evidence of localised inefficiencies. It should now be possible to carry out the same type of investigation on dyslexic readers who are older than the children in the normal sample and to draw conclusions as to which systems are impaired in each case and what types of strategic compensations have been adopted.

6 Dyslexic cases: Series I and II

6.1 The Tayside sample

In this and the two following chapters I will present the results of an application of the cognitive assessment procedure to the individual members of a sample of dyslexic subjects. The sample was recruited in the summer of 1981 and was based on contacts with educational psychologists, responses to a press announcement and liaison with a voluntary organisation, the Tayside Dyslexia Association.

The intention was to locate subjects who had histories of difficulty in learning to read and spell but who were of secondary school age or above and who had established at least a partial competence in reading. The group contained 24 members at the outset. Three of the older members were lost early on as a result of moves away from the district. This monograph will present information about the remaining 21 subjects who will be referred to as the 'Tayside sample'.

The approach to subject selection was open-ended. I did not consider that it was possible to define the characteristics to be met by a representative sample and did not wish to apply exclusionary criteria. (e.g. insistence on a particular IQ level) or to select subjects on some other basis, for example apparent similarity to cases of acquired dyslexia.

The sample is probably best defined simply as a group of individuals, resident in the Tayside area, whose problems in reading and spelling had been sufficient to trigger referral to the official agencies or the local voluntary organisation.

Table 6.1 identifies the 21 subjects by their initials and gives their ages at the time of recruitment (September 1981) and the results of an administration of the Schonell graded word tests of reading and spelling. An assessment of intellectual level, usually based on the Wechsler intelligence scales, is also given. If a report by an educational psychologist was available, and if this committed itself to a diagnostic opinion, then this has been indicated in the table.

TABLE 6.1 *Details of members of the Tayside dyslexic sample, including age in September 1981, Schonell reading and spelling ages in September 1981, and verbal and performance IQs determined by administration of the Wechsler tests. The cases are listed in their order of presentation in this and the following chapters*

Series	Case	Initials	Age	Wechsler		Schonell		Diagnosis
				VIQ	PIQ	RA	SA	
I	1	AD	17-7	106	132	12-6+	11-7	
	2	SS	25-3	125	130	12-6+	11-7	dysgraphia
	3	RO	16-10	126		12-6+	11-10	
	4	MF	14-8	106	126	12-3	11-11	weakness in auditory conceptualisation
II	1	FM	14-7	102	117	10-7	10-0	
	2	DP	16-1	104	114	12-2	11-7	STM impairment
	3	CE	13-0	114	106	11-10	10-0	auditory dyslexic
	4	DT	17-3	105	147	12-6+	12-1	
III	1	AR	14-6	117	121	11-0	10-4	visual dyslexia
	2	LA	12-11	122	118	11-6	8-8	auditory dyslexia
	3	SM	13-2	94	117	10-5	9-6	
	4	GS	13-5	121	83	9-9	8-5	
	5	LH	11-2	67	86	8-7	8-5	
IV	1	JM	14-2	112	90	11-4	10-8	
	2	SE	21-7	108	99	12-6+	7-11	difficulty with auditory conceptualisation
	3	MP	22-6	85	64	11-8	10-8	
V	1	SB	13-4	113	132	10-0	9-2	phonological difficulty
	2	LT	19-0	99	123	11-5	11-6	
	3	MT	14-11	100	107	12-2	8-1	
	4	JB	12-6	94	102	9-0	8-2	auditory difficulty
	5	PS	12-3	94	103	9-6	9-1	

The members of the sample undertook an extended version of the experimental series described in Chapter 4. The testing was carried out individually, using the Apple II microcomputer, in a quiet laboratory located in the Department of Psychology at the University of Dundee. The general procedure was the same as for the competent reader study regarding all such matters as the provision of practice, timing of displays, and the treatment of data. The subjects were paid for their participation on an hourly rate and any travel costs they incurred were refunded.

6.2   Preliminary classification of cases

Since the objective of the research was one of using the cognitive experimental procedures to establish descriptions of the processing systems of individual dyslexic subjects, it seemed appropriate that the results should be presented in the form of a series of case studies, each containing (1) a competence description, (2) a report on the results of the experiments, and (3) a 'cognitive description' stated within the terms of the information processing model. There are various ways in which such a series could be organised. The approach adopted in this instance was to treat each subject's efficiency in reading high frequency words as a primary dimension along which the cases could be ranked.

The presentation will, therefore, consist of a series of case studies which progresses from the subject who was most efficient in high frequency word reading to the subject who was most evidently impaired. Since an unbroken sequence of 21 case studies would be likely to prove indigestible, I have segmented the sequence into five sub-groups, each containing no more than 5 subjects. The identities of the subjects included in each sub-group are given in Table 6.1.

I would emphasise that this grouping is principally a matter of convenience of presentation. It does not reflect any presumptions about the existence or characteristics of dyslexic sub-types. The effect is that the subjects within a given sub-group will be likely to share approximately the same level of efficiency in the operation of route 'm' to phonology. The experimental analysis will indicate how their processing systems operated in the other domains. Contrasts between the descriptions of the members of each sub-group can then be considered in order to reach some preliminary conclusions about the questions of the homogeneity or heterogeneity of dyslexic impairments which were discussed earlier.

In this chapter I will present the results for the Series I and II subjects whose reading was relatively efficient. Chapters 7 and 8 will describe the data for subjects having more exaggerated morphemic or phonological impairments.

6.3 Series I case studies

I will start by presenting the cases of the four subjects whose high frequency word reading approximated most closely the performance of the competent readers discussed in Chapter 5. This group consisted of subjects AD, SS, RO and MF. All four were of above average ability and tended to emphasise spelling, not reading, as the main focus of their difficulties.

Case I.1   Andrew D (born March 1964)

1   Psycho-educational background

Andrew D was aged 17 years at the commencement of the project. He was then in his sixth year at secondary school and was studying Mathematics and Physics at CSYS level, Chemistry at the Higher Grade and Metalwork at 'O' Grade. In the previous year he had obtained SCE Higher Grade passes in Mathematics, Chemistry, Physics and Economics, but had failed English. He subsequently obtained a place at university and embarked on a degree course in science and engineering.

AD reported that his difficulties were in the area of spelling rather than reading and particularly concerned uncertainties about vowel combinations. He had been assessed by a neurologist at the age of 11 and was found to show superior ability in abstract non-verbal reasoning tasks but to have marked defects in writing and spelling. Weekly individual tuition was instituted and was maintained over a period of five years. He was permitted a concession of extra time in certain examinations.

An assessment by an educational psychologist at the age of 12 indicated a superior level of intelligence on the WISC performance scales (Performance IQ = 132, Verbal IQ = 106). Application of the Schonell graded word tests in 1981 gave a reading age of 12-6+ years and a spelling age of 11-7 years.

Note: References for tests used in the psycho-educational assessments appear in the bibliography on p. 260.

2   Experimental data

The experimental analysis of AD's reading functions confirmed that he was, in most respects, a normally competent reader. Results for vocalising high and low frequency words, shown in Table 6.2, fell well within the normal range. The reaction time distributions were well formed and contained no slow or outlying responses. There was a significant 35 ms effect of word frequency.

AD's reading of non-words, also shown in Table 6.2, was impaired with respect to accuracy (over 27 per cent of errors) but not reaction time. The main distribution of VRTs lay below 1750 ms and there were only a few slow responses within the range 2000-3000 ms. The lexicality effect of

TABLE 6.2   *Vocal reaction times (ms) and error rates for reading high frequency words, low frequency words and non-words by AD*

	High frequency words Overall Intercept Slope			Low frequency words Overall Intercept Slope			Non-words Overall Intercept Slope		
$\bar{\text{X}}$	723	626	20^1	758	618	31^1	1004	646	73^1
sd	150			188			395		
Error %	0.6			7.94			27.54		

[1] Linear trend significant at $p<0.05$ or better by F-test
Frequency effect: $t(281) = 1.726$, $p<0.05$. $\chi^2(1) = 10.744$, $p<0.01$
Lexicality effect (HF v NW): $t(336) = 8.576$, $p<0.001$. $\chi^2(1) = 52.14$, $p<0.001$
                        (LF v NW): $t(285) = 6.221$, $p=0.001$. $\chi^2(1) = 19.223$, $p<0.001$

267 ms was similar in magnitude to that shown by the competent readers who did not exhibit a phonological effect.

An analysis of AD's errors in non-word reading supported his own observation that complex vowels were a main cause of confusion. In the experiment varying vowel complexity he made 10 per cent of errors on non-words containing simple vowels as against 45 per cent on items containing complex vowels ($p<0.01$). The structural analysis of his error corpus indicated that complex vowels were correctly translated on only 8 per cent of occasions whereas his score was 61 per cent for simple vowels. Some errors illustrating AD's inaccuracy in vowel translation are: coist → 'coast', hool → 'hole', spaich → 'spatch'.

The accuracy of AD's word reading was not affected by form class, concrete/abstract meaning or spelling-to-sound irregularity. There was, however, a significant 76 ms effect of irregularity on the reaction time to read low frequency words.

AD's performance on the decision tasks was also proficient. In array matching, orthographically legal arrays were matched more than 200 ms faster than illegal arrays ($p<0.001$). Lexical decisions were made rapidly and accurately (RT = 730 ms, error rate = 6 per cent), and there were effects of frequency on positive RT and of legality on negative RT and accuracy. Semantic decision performance was well within the competent range (RT = 1045 ms, error = 7.63 per cent), although there were no significant effects of typicality or relatedness.

The analysis of AD's visual processor functions was also suggestive of normal functioning. The data from the matching experiments, summarised in Table 6.3, show fast and accurate performance which lies well within the range for the competent readers. The only features of note are the significant processing rates of 13-14 ms/letter in identity matching and evidence of a relatively fast left-to-right scan in the array matching tasks.

Table 6.2 also gives details of the effects of word length. The rates of 20-30 ms/letter for word reading and 73 ms/letter for non-word reading were significant on the linear trend test but fell within the normal range. Effects

TABLE 6.3   *Reaction times (ms) and error rates for visual matching tasks by AD for (1) standard experiment, (2) experiment varying format, and (3) experiment varying letter orientation*

Experiment		Identity matching Overall	Rate (ms/letter)	Array matching Overall	Position of difference (ms/position)
1	$\overline{X}$	657	13^1	$\overline{X}$ 1006	100^1
	sd	126		sd 297	
	Error %	2.5		Error % 6	
2	$\overline{X}$	705	14^1	$\overline{X}$ 1339	163^1
	sd	167		sd 411	
	Error %	3.7		Error % 6.67	
3	$\overline{X}$	543	-7	$\overline{X}$ 1450	44
	sd	127		sd 482	
	Error %	1.67		Error % 3.75	

[1] Linear trend significant at $p < 0.05$ or better by F-test

on lexical and semantic decision RTs were small and not significant. This suggests that AD's visual processor functioned normally in a parallel or fast serial mode. Results from the format distortion experiments have been summarised in Table 6.4. The distortion effects were appreciable in some instances, lying at about the upper end of the normal range, e.g. a rate of about 260 ms/letter for reading vertically distorted words.

TABLE 6.4   *Reaction times (ms) and error rates for reading normal and distorted words or non-words by AD*

		Vocalisation tasks Words	Non-words	Decision tasks Semantic	Lexical
Normal	$\overline{X}$	1055	1328	738	927
	sd	168	589	125	258
	Error %	0	40	4.17	0
	Rate	-3	-36	1	32
Zigzag	$\overline{X}$	1242^2	1462	858^2	1236^2
	sd	350	523	221	655
	Error %	3.33	26.67	2.08	3.33
	Rate	90^1	183^1	54^1	142^1
Vertical	$\overline{X}$	1658^2	1809^2	1003^2	1481^2
	sd	578	720	400	661
	Error %	6.67	46.67	0	5
	Rate	257^1	214	149^1	204^1

[1] Significant linear trend
[2] Format effect on reaction time
[3] Format effect on accuracy

Note: *The notes to tables have been done in a standard way. In some instances there will be no effects of the kind indicated by superscript numbers in the notes in that subject's data.*

3   Conclusions

AD's Level I (competence) description identifies him as a young man of superior scientific and non-verbal ability whose dyslexic problems relate to spelling rather than to reading.

The cognitive analysis of his reading functions suggests the presence of a 'phonological dyslexia' affecting the accuracy of grapheme-phoneme translation of complex vowel groups. An interpretation of his data, expressed in the terms of the processing model, might take the form shown in Table 6.5.

TABLE 6.5   *Summary of cognitive description of reading functions of subject AD*

Function	Status	Comment
'm' → phonology	Efficient	Small frequency effect. Grapheme-phoneme support for low frequency words
'g' → phonology	Impaired accuracy	Inaccurate on complex vowels
'm' → semantics	Efficient	Frequency effect
Visual processor	Efficient	Orthographic model

AD's results are similar to those of subject JK in the competent reader sample. They support the conclusion that route 'g' to phonology may be impaired in accuracy without there being a detectable effect on translation time. Further, liability to translation errors in route 'g' does not compromise the accuracy of route 'm' to phonology (or semantics). This dissociation provides evidence which may be used to argue in favour of the distinction between routes 'g' and 'm'.

Case I.2   Susan S (born May 1956)

1   Psycho-educational background

Susan S wrote in response to a press report about the project stating that she had experienced long-standing difficulties in spelling. She said that she had been brought up in New Zealand and had left school at an early age without taking any qualifications. She married at the age of 16 years and came to Britain. At the start of the project she was aged 25 years. She had a daughter aged 7 years and commented that she was worried that her child was also experiencing difficulty in acquiring basic reading and spelling competence. An assessment of her general abilities, using the Wechsler scales, indicated above average ability in both the verbal and the performance areas (full scale IQ = 128). Her score was at ceiling on the Schonell Graded Word Reading test. Her spelling age was 11-7 years.

2 Experimental data

Table 6.6 summarises the results for reading high frequency words, low frequency words and non-words. A plot of the reaction time distributions appears in Figure 6.1. Word reading was accurate. The reaction time levels were at the upper end of the competent reader range and the distributions were well formed. There was a significant word frequency effect of 87 ms. No morphemic impairment is suggested.

TABLE 6.6   *Vocal reaction times (ms) and error rates for reading high frequency words, low frequency words and non-words by SS*

| | High frequency words | | | Low frequency words | | | Non-words | | |
	Overall	Intercept	Slope	Overall	Intercept	Slope	Overall	Intercept	Slope
X̄	783	616	35[1]	869	750	25	1953	1126	169[1]
sd	179			245			1056		
Error %	1.2			8.8			23.83		

[1] Linear trend significant at p<0.05 or better by F-test
 Frequency effect: $t(277) = 3.361$, p<0.001. $\chi^2(1) = 9.713$, p<0.01
 Lexicality effect (HF v NW): $t(342) = 13.999$, p<0.001. $\chi^2(1) = 40.502$, p<0.001
  (LF v NW): $t(291) = 10.735$, p<0.001. $\chi^2(1) = 12.169$, p<0.001

There was a large effect of lexicality on error rate and reaction time. SS made 24 per cent of errors in non-word reading. The reaction time was slow at 1950 ms and widely dispersed with a distribution containing a preponderance of times below 2000 ms together with a substantial tail of slow outlying responses. The lexicality effect (the difference between non-words and low frequency words) was over 1000 ms. This slowness and inaccuracy in non-word reading is indicative of the presence of a phonological dyslexia (an impairment of route 'g' to phonology).

SS's word reading was not affected by the function/content distinction. However, abstract meaning slowed reactions to low frequency words by 100 ms or so (p<0.05). Spelling-to-sound irregularity increased error rate on low frequency words from 0 to 18.52 per cent (p<0.05) and produced a rise in VRT of about 50 ms (p<0.05). These results suggest an involvement of both semantic processing and grapheme-phoneme translation in word retrieval.

Non-word reading was not affected by homophony. An analysis of the results from the list in which the lexical environment of the non-words was manipulated indicated that only about 4 per cent of SS's responses were pronounced in accordance with larger (vowel + terminal consonant) correspondences. These data suggest that SS's grapheme-phoneme translator operated on primitive correspondences without reference to the vocabulary store.

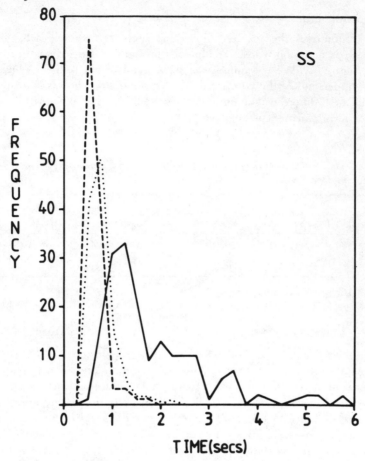

FIGURE 6.1   *Reaction time distributions for responses to high frequency words (– – –), low frequency words (. . .) and non-words (———) by subject SS*

TABLE 6.7   *Reaction time (ms) and error data for lexical and semantic decisions by SS*

	HF Words	LF Words	Lexical decisions Legal Non-words	Illegal Non-words	All
X	1013	1261²	2103²	1071	1252
sd	210	407	1062	267	627
Error %	0	0	5	0	0.83
Rate (ms/letter)		12	15	−53	−12

¹ Significant linear trend
² Significant effect on reaction time
³ Significant effect on error rate

SS made one derivational error (happen → 'happened') and two possible regularisation errors (corps → 'corpse', heir → 'hair'). The great majority of errors were minor failures of correspondence deriving from confusions over letter identities and positions. The responses were generally structurally close to the targets with more than 90 per cent having correspondence scores greater than 50 per cent. Translation accuracy was lower for vowels than for consonants, and for complex graphemes than for simple graphemes, ranging from 84 per cent correct for simple consonants to 26 per cent for complex vowels. An analysis of error reaction times indicated that non-word responses to non-words were made more slowly than word responses to word targets (1039 ms versus 2314 ms, p<0.01 by t-test). The error corpus included both word and non-word responses but gave no evidence of a bias in favour of one category or the other.

Table 6.7 summarises the results from the lexical and semantic decisions tasks. Semantic decisions were made accurately with a reaction within the range of the competent readers. Typicality had a significant effect on positive RT. Lexical decisions were also very accurate and were fast for all categories of item except the legal non-words. These responses, with a mean above 2000 ms, were significantly slower than responses to the illegal non-words. There was also an effect of word frequency of over 200 ms on positive reaction time. These results are not suggestive of any impairment of route 'm' to semantics. The delay in rejection of the legal non-words could reflect an involvement of SS's impaired grapheme-phoneme translator.

The results from the visual matching tasks appear in Table 6.8. Reaction times and error levels were well within the competent range and no general impairment of visual processor functions seems to be indicated. Legal arrays were matched 260 ms faster than illegal arrays (p<0.001). Length effects, summarised in Tables 6.6 and 6.7, were within the normal range for word reading and lexical and semantic decisions. The somewhat slower rate of 169 ms/letter observed for non-word reading is consistent with SS's

	Semantic decisions			
Typical positives	Atypical positives	Related negatives	Unrelated negatives	All
1039	1329[2]	1599	1854	1455
326	446	431	1460	875
0	0	6.67	0	1.69
				80

phonological dyslexia and suggests that her elevated reaction time is in part attributable to a tendency towards slow serial processing of non-words.

TABLE 6.8   *Reaction times (ms) and error rates for visual matching tasks by SS*

| | Identity matching | | | Array matching | |
	Overall	Rate (ms/letter)		Overall	Position of difference (ms/position)
$\overline{X}$	978	12	$\overline{X}$	1610	68
sd	222		sd	415	
Error %	1.67		Error %	3	

[1] Linear trend significant at p<0.05 or better by F-test

The effects of format distortions have been summarised in Table 6.9. The impact on lexical and semantic decisions was no greater than that observed in the competent reader sample. In the vocalisation tasks the processing rates for non-word reading were extremely slow, suggesting that the distortions may have exaggerated an existing tendency to process these items serially. Processing rates for distorted words were also slower than 300 ms/letter for zigzag high frequency words and vertical low frequency words. It seems possible that route 'm' to phonology was more vulnerable to disruption by distortion than route 'm' to semantics. Aside from this, the data suggest that SS's visual processor functions were unimpaired.

TABLE 6.9   *Reaction times (ms) and error rates for reading normal and distorted words or non-words by SS*

| | Vocalisation tasks | | Decision tasks | |
	Words	Non-words	Semantic	Lexical
Normal $\overline{X}$	1017	1800	898	1138
sd	606	855	384	696
Error %	3.33	23.33	0	3.33
Rate	172[1]	264[1]	36	149[1]
Zigzag $\overline{X}$	1373[2]	2094	1040	1469[1]
sd	551	893	330	682
Error %	3.33	33.33	0	3.33
Rate	169[1]	314[1]	69[1]	87
Vertical $\overline{X}$	1689[2]	2927[2]	1176[2]	1535[2]
sd	944	1805	451	601
Error%	3.33	26.67	0	3.33
Rate	180	543[1]	159[1]	154[1]

[1] Significant linear trend
[2] Format effect on reading time
[3] Format effect on accuracy

3 Conclusions

SS's Level I (competence) description is very incomplete and does not go much beyond the observation that she is an intelligent young woman of limited formal education whose dyslexic problems relate to spelling more obviously than to reading.

The Level II (cognitive) analysis of her reading functions is indicative of the presence of a 'phonological dyslexia' affecting both the accuracy and the speed of grapheme-phoneme translation. Table 6.10 gives a summary of the conclusions from the experimental data stated within the terms of the four domains of the information processing model. Taken in conjunction with the results of the normal readers and subject AD this description supports the conclusion that route 'g' to phonology may be impaired with respect to accuracy, translation time, or both. SS's data offer a further demonstration that an impairment of route 'g' need not compromise the operations of the morphemic routes to phonology or semantics. Some justification for the distinction between the two morphemic routes is offered by the differential effects of format distortion on performance in the vocalisation and decision tasks.

TABLE 6.10 *Summary of cognitive description of reading functions of subject SS*

Function	Status	Comment
'm' → phonology	Efficient	Frequency effect. Semantic and grapheme-phoneme support for low frequency words
'g' → phonology	Impaired	Inaccurate on complex vowels. Simple correspondences. No lexical support. Serial processing. Slow translation
'm' → semantics	Efficient	Frequency effect. Typicality effect
Visual processor	Efficient	Orthographic model. Slow format resolution for non-words

Case I.3   Richard O (born December 1964)

1   Psycho-educational background

Richard O was born in England and lived there until he was aged about 7 years. His language development was considered to have been delayed and his early speech to have been very indistinct. A hearing test administered at 4 years revealed slightly defective hearing which improved following the removal of his tonsils and adenoids. There were also reports of clumsiness and poor co-ordination. After his family had moved to Scotland his reading development was found to lag behind that of his classmates but he apparently responded well to teaching. A lisp was noticed by a speech therapist and some corrective instruction was given. After transferring to secondary school, RO was referred to the area educational psychologist because his teachers considered that his attainment fell short of his ability. The psychologist reported that he had good verbal intelligence but that his written work appeared dysgraphic. In 1977 a further assessment was undertaken by the Tayside Dyslexia Association. This confirmed that RO's intelligence was well above average and suggested that he was a competent reader with a marked spelling disability. His WISC IQ was estimated at 128 and he was found to be at age or above on the Neale reading test but to be about 3 years behind his age on the Daniels and Diack spelling test. The psychologist noted a slight impairment of auditory discrimination, assessed by the Wepman test, and commented on RO's mixed dominance (left eye dominant but right hand and foot) and difficulties in sequencing. A dysgraphia and a specific spelling deficit were diagnosed. An assessment in 1981, using the Schonell graded word tests, gave a reading age at ceiling and a spelling age of 11-10 years. Despite his background of difficulties, RO passed three subjects at 'O' Grade in his fourth year at secondary school and a further five subjects the next year. He went on to obtain passes in Chemistry, Geography, English and Biology at the Higher Grade.

2 Experimental data

RO's results for reading high frequency words, low frequency words and non-words appear in Table 6.11. The distributions of vocal reaction times have been plotted in Figure 6.2. Words were very accurately read with reaction times falling into a well-formed distribution with a mean just above the range for the competent readers. There was a 44 ms effect of word frequency. These data are indicative of an efficient morphemic route to phonology. Form class, abstract meaning and spelling-to-sound irregularity did not exert significant effects on either accuracy or vocal reaction time.

TABLE 6.11 *Vocal reaction times (ms) and error rates for reading high frequency words, low frequency words and non-words by RO*

| | High frequency words | | | Low frequency words | | | Non-words | | |
	Overall	Intercept	Slope	Overall	Intercept	Slope	Overall	Intercept	Slope
$\bar{X}$	838	711	26[1]	882	784	21	1336	249	221[1]
sd	142			203			580		
Error %	1.2			3.2			4.66		

[1] Linear trend significant at $p<0.05$ or better by F-test
  Frequency effect: $t(284) = 2.144$, $p = 0.025$. $\chi^2(1) = 1.424$
  Lexicality effect (HF v NW): $t(388) = 10.76$, $p = 0.001$. $\chi^2(1) = 3.758$
                    (LF v NW): $t(454) = 8.311$, $p = 0.001$. $\chi^2(1) < 1$

Non-words were accurately read with a latency at about the level identified with a mild phonological effect in the results of the competent readers. The lexicality effect, at 454 ms, was somewhat exaggerated and the

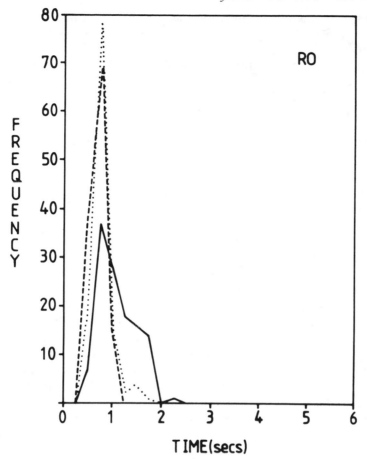

FIGURE 6.2 *Reaction time distributions for responses to high frequency words (– – –), low frequency words (. . .) and non-words (———) by RO*

distribution, although overlapping the data for words and quite well formed, was relatively widely dispersed. Non-word homophony did not have consistent effects on accuracy or VRT. Only a minority of responses to non-words (about 5 per cent) gave evidence of the use of V+C correspondences. Error responses were generally structurally similar to the targets (average similarity score = 74 per cent).

Table 6.12 contains a summary of the results from the decision tasks. Semantic decisions were accurate and fast. There was a 476 ms effect of negative relatedness. Lexical decisions were also efficiently made and showed a strong effect of orthographic legality on negative reaction time. These data suggest efficient functioning of route 'm' to semantics.

The results from the various visual matching experiments appear in Table 6.13. Identity matching was accurately achieved with reaction times

TABLE 6.12   *Reaction time (ms) and error data for lexical and semantic decisions by RO*

		HF Words	LF Words	Lexical decisions Legal Non-words	Illegal Non-words	All
	$\bar{X}$	802	770	1325[2]	965	938
	sd	159	172	430	253	316
Error %		2.63	18.18[3]	10	0	5.83
Rate (ms/letter)			31	−54	17	14

[1] Significant linear trend
[2] Significant effect on reaction time
[3] Significant effect on error rate

which, at 1200-1300 ms, lay at the upper bound of the competent range. Analyses of the effects of variations in display size revealed an unusually large impact (76 ms/letter in one experiment, 90 ms/letter for responses to vertically formatted displays in a second). Array matching, although accurate, involved an extreme elevation of the RT to 2500-3000 ms. These values are well above those of any of the competent readers, including the two subjects who were thought to show a mild visual processor effect and are suggestive of a visual processor impairment possibly affecting the capacity of the processor to operate in analytic mode on the letter arrays. RO showed a large effect of orthographic legality (over 600 ms). In the standard array matching experiment there was no clear evidence of left-to-

TABLE 6.13   *Reaction times (ms) and error rates for visual matching tasks*

Experiment		Identity matching Overall	Rate (ms/letter)		Array matching Overall	Position of difference (ms/position)
1	$\bar{X}$	1281	54[1]	$\bar{X}$	2545	103
	sd	388		sd	736	
	Error %	2.5		Error %	2	
2	$\bar{X}$	1363	61[1]	$\bar{X}$	3032	324[1]
	sd	398		sd	995	
	Error %	0.62		Error %	2.5	
3	$\bar{X}$	1053	7	$\bar{X}$	2544	209[1]
	sd	247		sd	780	
	Error %	0		Error %	0.63	

[1] Linear trend significant at p<0.05 or better by F-test

		Semantic decisions		
Typical positives	Atypical positives	Related negatives	Unrelated negatives	All
1216	1127	1868	1392[2]	1395
335	291	929	500	631
0	6.67	6.9	0	3.39
				73[1]

right processing. However, the position of difference functions for the two subsidiary experiments had slopes of about 300 ms/position, again somewhat slower than those shown by competent readers who used a serial self-terminating procedure in matching.

Further information about RO's visual processor functions can be obtained by considering the effects of word length and format distortion. The length effects have been included in Tables 6.11 and 6.12. The effect on vocalisation of high frequency words (26 ms/letter) was close to the range of the competent readers. There were no clear effects on lexical decision RT and the rate of 76 ms/letter observed for semantic decisions was within the normal range. These results suggest that the visual processing underlying the operation of the morphemic routes was normal. Non-word reading, by contrast, involved a processing rate of 221 ms/letter. This rate is substantially slower than those of the competent readers who did not show phonological effects. One possibility is that non-word reading is more obviously dependent on analytic processing than word reading and hence more sensitive to an impairment of the analytic mode.

This speculation has implications for the kinds of results which might be expected from the format distortion experiments. A general trend in the competent reader sample was for distortion to produce a slowing of the time per letter index. It was suggested that this might be because the resolution of the distortion required an analytic operation on the letter array. If RO has a visual processor impairment which affects speed of analytic processing, then it follows that he should have particular difficulty with the distortions. The data summarised in Table 6.14 suggest that this prediction can be supported for the reading of the vertical format. In the word vocalisation experiments processing rates approximated 600 ms/letter. Rates above 400 ms/letter were observed for the non-word reading task and in the lexical and semantic decision experiments. These processing rates lie well outside the range of the competent readers.

TABLE 6.14   *Reaction times (ms) and error rates for reading normal and distorted words or non-words by RO*

		Vocalisation tasks		Decision tasks	
		Words	Non-words	Semantic	Lexical
Normal	X̄	946	1318	1222	1585
	sd	324	481	342	739
Error %		0	16.67	2.08	1.67
	Rate	52	164[1]	69[1]	259[1]
Zigzag	X̄	1149[2]	1809[2]	1571[2]	2058[2]
	sd	374	645	683	1097
Error%		3.33	6.67	0	5
	Rate	36	215[1]	122	427[1]
Vertical	X̄	2113[2]	2400[2]	2463[2]	3381[2]
	sd	1814	1086	1612	2290
Error %		10	6.67	2.17	5
	Rate	604[1]	542[1]	573[1]	462[1]

[1] Significant linear trend
[2] Format effect on reaction time
[3] Format effect on accuracy

3   Conclusions

The Level I (competence) account of RO's case suggests that he shares with AD and SS the features of being an individual of above average ability whose dyslexic problems are considered to affect spelling rather than reading. An earlier history of impaired speech perception and production was also indicated.

From the Level II (cognitive) analysis it is clear that his reading processes were different from those of AD and SS, and that the predominant feature was a 'visual processor dyslexia' possibly affecting the analytic processing mode. A cognitive description, formulated by reference to the domains of the processing model, can be proposed along the lines suggested in Table 6.15. A first conclusion to be drawn from RO's data is that a visual processor impairment may be identified as an alternative to the phonological effects evident in the results of AD and SS. In RO's case, as in the milder examples found in the competent reader example, the visual processor defect appeared not to compromise the operation of the morphemic routes to phonology and semantics. One possibility is that morpheme recognition depends on wholistic (or segmental) visual processing, and that this function is distinct from the analytic process required for point-by-point comparison or format distortion resolution. The proposal that the *analytic mode* was impaired in RO's case while the wholistic mode remained efficient is consistent with the observation that length effects were slight in the word reading tasks but quite substantial in the non-word reading tasks, where analytic processing may be required to isolate

TABLE 6.15   *Summary of cognitive description of reading functions of subject RO*

Function	Status	Comment
'm' → phonology	Efficient	Frequency effect
'g' → phonology	Efficient	Slow serial processing
'm' → semantics	Efficient	Relatedness effect
Visual processor	Impaired	Orthographic model. Slow processing rates in identity matching. Very slow responses in array matching. Serial processing. Very slow resolution of vertical distortions

particular graphemes. According to this argument, slow serial processing in non-word reading should be a usual accompaniment of an impaired analytic function indexed by slow matching and format resolution.

Some commentators (e.g. Frith, 1985) have argued that a dyslexic pattern in which competent reading is accompanied by poor spelling might derive from an inability to attend analytically to orthographic detail. It might, on this hypothesis, be suggested that RO's poor spelling was a consequence of his impaired analytic function. However, such a conclusion appears not to be warranted, since AD and SS showed a good reader/poor speller pattern in the context of another type of impairment, while the competent readers LH and LL exhibited slowness of visual matching in the absence of an effect on spelling.

Case I.4   Morag F (born December 1966)

1   Psycho-educational background

Morag F's mother, a teacher in special education, wrote in response to a press report on the project to comment that her younger daughter, then aged 14 years, had exhibited a particular difficulty in spelling. This was confirmed by an examination of her school books which contained numerous phonetically accurate mis-spellings.

Morag's birth was reported to have been normal and there was no family history of learning disability. Between 6 and 13 weeks of age she was hospitalised on account of broncho-pneumonia. Early onset of speech was said to have been delayed and confusion over the order of sounds in words was noted. Motor development was normal and no particular problems with learning to tie shoelaces or to read the clock were reported. Her mother suspected learning difficulties from the age of about 5 years and arranged for individual help. Morag appears to have maintained a positive attitude to school. She passed four subjects at the Higher Grade (Mathematics, Physics, Chemistry and English) and proceeded to a College of Art with the aim of following a degree course in interior design. Her hobbies are sport, sewing and drawing. She still dislikes reading and does not read for pleasure.

An assessment of her general intelligence was made early in 1985 using the WAIS. A summary of the scaled scores appears in Table 6.16. These indicate an average level of verbal ability, with depression on the digit span sub-test, combined with above average performance abilities. An evident difficulty with the arithmetic sub-test and a slowness in giving vocabulary definitions attracted comment.

TABLE 6.16   *Results of administration of the WAIS to subject MF in 1985*

Verbal tests		Performance tests	
Information	10	Digit symbol	14
Comprehension	12	Picture completion	15
Arithmetic	10	Block design	15
Similarities	11	Picture arrangement	13
Digit span	8	Object assembly	12
Vocabulary	10		
Verbal IQ	106	Performance IQ	126

In 1981 MF's reading age on the Schonell test was 12-3 years. Comprehension tests, administered in 1985, gave a score of 13-7 years on the Daniels and Diack untimed test and of 11-6 years on the Schonell timed test. It was suggested that discrepancy reflected the slowness of her reading. Her score on the Schonell spelling test was 11-11 years in 1981 and had risen to 12-8 years in 1985. Her handwriting was described as satisfactory but with poor punctuation, capitalisation and spelling. A difficulty with consonant doubling was noted.

There was no indication of visual impairment. Her score on the Graham Kendall Memory for Designs test was normal and orthopotics testing showed a fixed reference eye and no visual anomalies. On the Lindamood Auditory Conceptualisation test her score was 88/100 which was described as indicative of some weakness in the ability to reflect on the identity, number and sequence of sounds in words. Nonsense word reading was efficient (20/22 correct).

2   Experimental data

Table 6.17 summarises the results for reading high frequency words, low frequency words and non-words. The vocal reaction time distributions appear in Figure 6.3. Word reading was very accurate and the reaction time distributions were well formed with a mean slightly above the level of the competent reader sample. There was a somewhat exaggerated word frequency effect (over 200 ms). The effects of form class, abstract meaning and spelling-to-sound irregularity were not significant. This suggests that

TABLE 6.17   *Vocal reaction times (ms) and error rates for reading high frequency words, low frequency words and non-words by MF*

| | High frequency words | | | Low frequency words | | | Non-words | | |
	Overall	Intercept	Slope	Overall	Intercept	Slope	Overall	Intercept	Slope
$\bar{X}$	932	670	55[1]	1141	782	77[1]	1743	447	266[1]
sd	337			516			1063		
Error %	1.19			3.17			8.9		

[1] Linear trend significant at p<0.05 or better by F-test
Frequency effect: t(286) = 4.132, p<0.001. $\chi^2(1)$ = 1.418
Lexicality effect (HF v NW):t(379) = 9.44,   p<0.001. $\chi^2(1)$ = 10.86, p<0.001
                  (LF v NW):t(335) = 5.854, p<0.001. $\chi^2(1)$ = 4.186, p<0.05

words were read by a direct process without the support of concurrent semantic processing or grapheme-phoneme translation.

Non-word reading was accurate but the reaction time was elevated and the distribution was dispersed and included a number of slow responses. The lexicality effect, at over 600 ms, was somewhat exaggerated. A mild phonological impairment is indicated.

Non-word reading was not affected by homophony. The errors were generally structurally close to the target (average similarity = 72 per cent) with complex vowel clusters the main focus of error. Three errors were considered to be phonetic regularisations (agility pronounced with a hard 'g', come → 'comb', below → 'bellow'). The others involved minor confusions and mis-translations (paunch → 'punch', dive → 'drive', drap → 'drab', scraim → 'scream', thrish → 'thirst'). Only about 4 per cent of responses to non-words made use of higher order correspondences. These data suggest that MF's translator operated on simple grapheme-phoneme correspondences without reference to the speech production lexicon.

Table 6.18 contains a summary of the results from the lexical and semantic decision experiments. Semantic decisions were made with a reaction time and error level which lay at the upper boundary of the range for the competent readers. There were large effects of typicality and relatedness (the typicality effect was more than 700 ms). The reaction time distribution was widely dispersed over the intervals 500 ms to 3500 ms. Lexical decisions were very accurate and were made with a reaction time which lay just above the normal range. The distribution was well formed with a majority of responses below 2000 ms. There was a 160 ms effect of word frequency on positive RT and a 600 ms effect of legality on negative RT. It seems that the morphemic route to semantics might reasonably be described as efficient although this conclusion is subject to the qualification that the reaction time levels were somewhat high and the psycholinguistic effects somewhat exaggerated.

The results from the visual matching experiments have been summarised

TABLE 6.18   *Reaction time (ms) and error data for lexical and semantic decisions by MF*

		HF Words	LF Words	Lexical decisions Legal Non-words	Illegal Non-words	All
	X̄	974	1134[2]	1627	1037[2]	1125
	sd	294	375	587	289	429
Error %		0	9.09	10	0	3.33
Rate (ms/letter)			18	377[1]	85[1]	100[1]

[1] Significant linear trend
[2] Significant effect on reaction time
[3] Significant effect on error rate

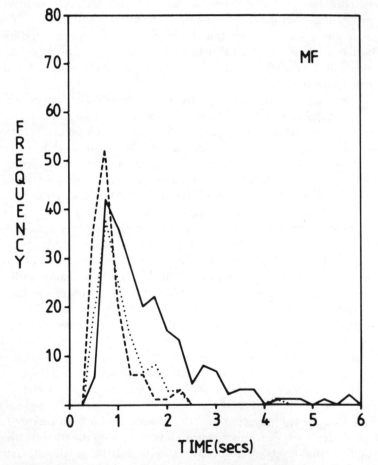

FIGURE 6.3   *Reaction time distributions for reading high frequency words (– – –), low frequency words (. . .) and non-words (———) by subject MF*

Typical positives	Atypical positives	Semantic decisions Related negatives	Unrelated negatives	All
1118	1843[2]	2120	1678[2]	1673
487	772	802	586	762
3.45	13.79	16.67	6.67	10.17
				131[1]

in Table 6.19. Identity matching was accurate and the reaction time was within but near the upper boundary of the normal range. Reaction time in array matching was high at over 2000 ms and there was evidence of serial left-to-right processing with a rate of 150-250 ms/position. There was a 300 ms effect of orthographic legality on positive RT.

TABLE 6.19 *Reaction times (ms) and error rates for visual matching tasks by MF*

Experiment		Identity matching Overall	Rate (ms/letter)		Array matching Overall	Position of difference (ms/position)
1	$\overline{X}$	1107	28[1]	$\overline{X}$	2139	153[1]
	sd	367		sd	667	
	Error %	0.83		Error %	0	
2	$\overline{X}$	1239	−2	$\overline{X}$	1714	241[1]
	sd	475		sd	613	
	Error %	1.23		Error %	3.33	
3	$\overline{X}$	887	8	$\overline{X}$	2065	155[1]
	sd	355		sd	618	
	Error %	0		Error %	3.13	

[1] Linear trend significant at $p < 0.05$ or better by F-test

The elevation of MF's reaction times in the array matching tasks suggests the possibility of an impairment of the analytic function of the visual processor of the kind shown by RO. This is supported by the findings from the format distortion experiments which appear in Table 6.20. In the vocalisation and decision tasks processing rates for reading vertically distorted words were extremely slow, often exceeding 400 ms/letter. These rates lay well outside the range observed for the competent readers.

TABLE 6.20   *Reaction times (ms) and error rates for reading normal and distorted words or non-words by MF*

		Vocalisation tasks		Decision tasks	
		Words	Non-words	Words	Non-words
Normal	X̄	1422	1793	1588	1414
	sd	932	971	644	636
Error %		3.45	23.33	2.17	3.33
	Rate	299[1]	261[1]	78	53
Zigzag	X̄	1622	2187	1838	1740[2]
	sd	801	1027	941	638
Error %		0	3.33[3]	2.08	5
	Rate	306[1]	367[1]	125	148[1]
Vertical	X̄	2178[2]	2524[2]	2454[2]	2153[2]
	sd	1485	1095	1266	751
Error %		3.33	13.33	10.42	6.67
	Rate	511[1]	358[1]	482[1]	293[1]

[1] Significant linear trend
[2] Format effect on reaction time
[3] Format effect on accuracy

In RO's case the analytic impairment appeared to exaggerate the effects of length in non-word reading but not in word reading. MF's processing rates for the vocalisation and decision tasks have been included in Tables 6.17 and 6.18. The rate of 266 ms/letter observed for non-word reading was exaggerated relative to the results of competent readers who did not show phonological effects. The effect also occurred in responses to legal non-words in the lexical decision experiment (rate = 377 ms/letter). It contrasts with the results for word reading (55 ms/letter for vocalising high frequency words, 18 ms/letter for positive responses in the lexical decision task). The rate for semantic decisions was slower but within the range of the competent readers.

3   Conclusions

MF's Level I (competence) description defines her as a young woman of above average non-verbal abilities and good motor skill whose dyslexic difficulties lie in the area of spelling rather than reading. Mild problems relating to speech development, production and conceptualisation are also indicated.

The Level II (cognitive) description identifies a 'visual processor dyslexia' as the predominant features, although there are hints of some accompanying mild phonological and morphemic effects. Table 6.21 gives a summary of the cognitive interpretation of MF's results. This description is similar to the one proposed for subject RO. The principal difference between the two cases is that MF shows some effects on the morphemic routes which are not evident in RO's data. These include a tendency towards serial processing and an enlargement of effects indexing semantic and phonological retrieval. One possibility is that these reflect general properties of MF's semantic processor and tap the same features as gave rise to the verbal-performance discrepancy on the WAIS (about 20 points of IQ) and produced the hesitations in verbal retrieval which were noted by the educational psychologist.

TABLE 6.21   *Summary of cognitive description of reading functions of subject MF*

Function	Status	Comment
'm' → phonology	Efficient	Frequency effect
'g' → phonology	Mild effect on latency	Serial processing. Simple correspondences
'm' → semantics	Mild effect on decision time	Frequency effect. Enlarged typicality and relatedness effects
Visual processor	Impaired	Orthographic model. Slow array matching. Serial processing. Very slow format resolution

Conclusions: Series I

Each of the four subjects included in this first sub-group exhibits a distinctive processing configuration. Nonetheless, it seems possible to conclude that two of the subjects, AD and SS, are characterised by a 'phonological dyslexia' whereas the other two give evidence of a 'visual analytic dyslexia'.

There were differences between the two phonological cases. AD's reading functions were in general not distinguishable from those of a normally competent reader. Inaccuracy of translation, particularly of graphemically complex vowels, was the only dyslexic feature. In SS's case, there were effects on both the accuracy and the rate of functioning of route 'g', and evidence for support of word retrieval by semantic processing in addition to grapheme-phoneme translation.

Differences were also evident between Cases I.3 and I.4. RO's reading was efficient for both words and non-words. Aside from the slow processing rate in non-word reading, the principal dyslexic features were processing delays in visual matching and format distortion resolution. MF exhibited similar visual processor effects, but showed in addition some evidence of

TABLE 6.22   *Results of administration of tests to subject FM (a) when subject's CA was*

	IQ scores	
	WISC-R:	
	full	110
	verbal	102
a	performance	117
	British Ability Scale:	
	matrices:	113
	information processing:	144
b		

delays affecting semantic and phonological retrieval.

These results argue against the hypothesis that all dyslexic cases are likely to receive similar cognitive descriptions. The differences between AD and SS, and between RO and MF, also emphasise the inadvisability of resorting too quickly to interpretations which assume the existence of a small number of dyslexic configurations or sub-types.

6.4 Series II case studies

The second sub-group of subjects also consisted of four members, FM, DP, CE and DT. Two of them, FM and CE, were younger than the subjects so far considered. CE shared with the Series I subjects a diagnosis which emphasised spelling difficulties as being more critical than reading difficulties.

Case II.1   Fiona M (born January 1967)

1   Psycho-educational background

Fiona's birth was described as 'at risk' and was induced at 7 months on account of maternal illness. In 1980, when she was in her first year at secondary school, her mother reported that she had problems with reading, spelling and pronouncing words, that she had earlier produced mirror writing, and that her current difficulties at school and with her homework were adversely affecting her general behaviour.

An intellectual assessment using an abbreviated WISC gave the scaled scores shown in Table 6.22. These indicate an above average IQ level combined with a depression on the digit span sub-test. Table 6.22 also gives details of results from reading and spelling tests. Reading comprehension appears only slightly retarded but FM was well behind her age on the rate

12-11 years and (b) when subject's CA (chronological age) was 14-8 years

Reading ages			Spelling ages	
Neale Analysis			Daniels and Diack	
rate	9-1 years		(test 11)	
accuracy	9-7 years		9-8 years	
comprehension	12-0 years			
Daniels and Diack (test 12)	11-2 years			
Schonell:	11-5 years		Schonell:	10-0 years

and accuracy measures and in spelling.

Administration of the Wepman Auditory Discrimination test gave indications of confusions over the phonemes /f/, /v/ and /m/. Writing was said to be immature in form, poor in spelling and limited in quantity of output but with good ideas and satisfactory sentence structure. The psychologist concluded that FM was a girl of above average ability who had a specific problem in reading and spelling combined with a short-term memory deficit. One-to-one tuition was recommended. Arrangements were made with a teacher who lived locally and a period of intensive tuition was ended after about six months on account of Fiona's excellent progress.

2   Experimental data

Table 6.23 gives details of the accuracy and reaction time data obtained from the vocalisation experiment. The reaction time distributions are shown in Figure 6.4. High frequency words were accurately read with a reaction time which, at over 1000 ms, lay slightly above the competent reader range. The distribution was dispersed and included two outliers. These indications of a morphemic impairment were reinforced by the data for low frequency word reading. The error level, at 20 per cent, was well

TABLE 6.23   *Vocal reaction times (ms) and error rates for reading high frequency words, low frequency words and non-words by FM*

	High frequency words			Low frequency words			Non-words		
	Overall	Intercept	Slope	Overall	Intercept	Slope	Overall	Intercept	Slope
X̄	1087	441	136[1]	1456	515	203[1]	2607	−343	621[1]
sd	484			781			1594		
Error %	2.38			19.84			22.13		

[1] Linear trend significant at p<0.05 or better by F-test

Frequency effect: t(263) = 4.727, p.<0.001. $\chi^2(1)$ = 24.688, p<0.001

Lexicality effect (HF v NW):t(345) = 11.696, p.<0.001. $\chi^2(1)$ = 31.927, p<0.001

(LF v NW):t(282) = 6.792, p<0.001. $\chi^2(1)$ = 0.256

above the range for the competent readers and the reaction time distribution included a substantial tail of slow responses. The frequency effect of over 300 ms was also exaggerated.

Non-words were read with a relatively high error rate (22 per cent) and with a slow reaction time (over 2600 ms). The vocal reaction time distribution included numerous slow responses with values up to 5000 ms and above. The difference between non-words and low frequency words was not significant for error rate but there was a large effect (1150 ms) on reaction time. These results are indicative of a phonological impairment.

FM's word reading was not affected by the function/content distinction or by abstract meaning, but there was an effect of over 300 ms of spelling-to-sound irregularity on reaction time to read low frequency words (p<0.05). This suggests that word retrieval was supported by grapheme-phoneme translation but not by semantic processing. There was an effect of non-word homophony on error rate in non-word reading but not on reaction time.

Error responses were generally structurally close to the target. Only 8 per cent of errors had similarity scores of less than 50 per cent (average = 67 per cent). Simple graphemes were more accurately translated than complex clusters (76 per cent of correct correspondences for simple consonants as against 28 per cent for complex vowels). FM's error responses were words and non-words with approximately equal frequencies. The errors were a mixture of visual confusions (wicked → 'winked', ewe → 'eve', canoe → 'canon'), derivational errors (variety → 'varied', beauty → 'beautiful', aisle → 'aisles') and phonetic regularisations (heir → 'hair', ski → 'sky', debt → 'dept'). Letter omissions and additions appeared to underlie many of the errors.

Table 6.24 summarises the results from the lexical and semantic decisions tasks. Semantic decisions were accurately made but the reaction time level was somewhat above the competent reader range and the distribution was widely dispersed and included some very slow responses. There was a large effect of typicality on positive reaction time and an effect of negative relatedness on accuracy. Lexical decisions were accurate for responses to words and illegal non-words but subject to numerous errors in classification of legal non-words (over 60 per cent). There was a large effect of frequency on positive reaction time (almost 400 ms). Negative responses were somewhat slow for illegal non-words and extremely elevated for the few legal non-words which were correctly classified. This poor discrimination in lexical decisions combined with the slow responses in the semantic decision task is suggestive of an effect on the morphemic route to semantics.

FM therefore gives a clearer indication than any of the subjects so far considered of the presence of a morphemic impairment affecting the routes to phonology and semantics. One possibility, discussed by Seymour and MacGregor (1984), is that this type of impairment derives from a disorder

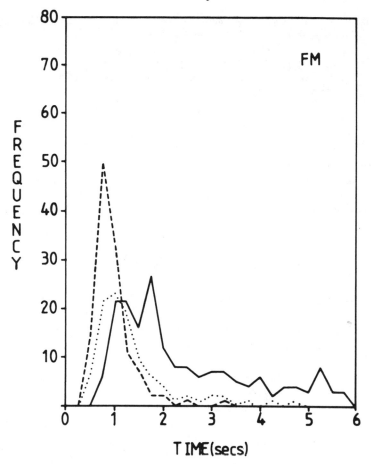

FIGURE 6.4 *Reaction time distributions for responses to high frequency words (– – –), low frequency words (. . .) and non-words (———) by FM*

of the wholistic function of the visual processor. It would then be expected that word reading should give evidence of serial processing marked by a strong linear relationship between reaction time and word length.

The slopes of the lines fitted to the data from the vocalisation and decision tasks appear in Tables 6.23 and 6.24. Responses to words involved a slow serial process in all instances except positive lexical decisions. The rates of 250 ms/letter observed for semantic decisions, and of 130-200 ms/letter for word reading, lie outside the range found in the competent reader sample. In order to reduce the contribution of outlying responses the data for word vocalisation were reanalysed with reaction times greater than 3000 ms removed. This reduced the slope values to about 100 ms/letter, although the linear trend remained strongly significant. Processing rates in

TABLE 6.24   *Reaction time (ms) and error data for lexical and semantic decisions by FM*

		HF Words	LF Words	Lexical decisions Legal Non-words	Illegal Non-words	All
	$\bar{X}$	994	1392[2]	4727	1446[2]	1522
	sd	262	409	2304	662	1226
Error %		0	0.09	60[3]	0	11.67
Rate (ms/letter)		68		960	209[1]	125

[1] Significant linear trend
[2] Significant effect on reaction time
[3] Significant effect on error rate

non-word reading were considerably slower (over 600 ms/letter).

Table 6.25 summarises the results from the visual matching tasks. These data contrast with the results of RO and MF in that they do not give evidence of a general impairment of the visual processor. The reaction time and accuracy for both tasks were well within the competent reader range. There was no clear evidence of serial processing in the array matching task and no significant effects of orthographic legality.

TABLE 6.25   *Reaction times (ms) and error rates for visual matching tasks by FM*

Experiment		Identity matching Overall	Rate (ms/letter)		Array matching Overall	Position of difference (ms/position)
1	$\bar{X}$	826	20[1]	$\bar{X}$	1321	77
	sd	238		sd	406	
	Error %	1.67		Error %	2	
2	$\bar{X}$	955	29[1]	$\bar{X}$	1873	28
	sd	350		sd	557	
	Error %	0.62		Error %	1.67	
3	$\bar{X}$	767	12[1]	$\bar{X}$	1619	70
	sd	212		sd	451	
	Error %	0		Error %	1.25	

[1] Linear trend significant at $p<0.05$ or better by F-test

The format distortion effects are documented in Table 6.26. It is clear that FM was considerably affected by distortion. In word reading her rates for processing vertical displays exceeded 500-600 ms/letter. Rates of well over 300 ms/letter occurred in the semantic and lexical decision tasks. In

Typical positives	Atypical positives	Semantic decisions Related negatives	Unrelated negatives	All
1561	2503[2]	2353	2468	2201
805	1533	631	1484	1241
0	11.11	13.33[3]	0	5.98
				249[1]

TABLE 6.26   *Reaction times (ms) and error rates for reading normal and distorted words or non-words by FM*

		Vocalisation tasks Words	Non-words	Decision tasks Semantic	Lexical
Normal	$\bar{\text{X}}$	1373	2523	1669	2885
	sd	460	914	939	2177
Error %		3.33	13.33	6.38	6.67
	Rate	65	274[1]	237[1]	53
Zigzag	$\bar{\text{X}}$	1691	2818	2122[2]	3747[2]
	sd	936	1415	1348	2709
Error %		6.67	16.67	4.26	11.67
	Rate	293[1]	511[1]	434[1]	244
Vertical	$\bar{\text{X}}$	2143[2]	2931	2191[2]	4574[2]
	sd	1139	1408	1385	3220
Error %		13.33	20	6.25	8.33
	Rate	583[1]	710[1]	389[1]	492

[1] Significant linear trend
[2] Format effect on reaction time
[3] Format effect on accuracy

non-word reading distortion appeared greatly to exaggerate an already slow and serial process.

3   Conclusions

FM's Level I (competence) description identifies her as a girl of above average ability who has difficulty in reading and spelling. The possibility of accompanying defects in auditory discrimination and verbal short-term memory is also indicated.

The Level II (cognitive) description, summarised in Table 6.27, suggests that her reading was subject to a number of impairments. This configuration differs from the interpretation assigned to any of the cases so far considered. FM exhibits a phonological dyslexia affecting both translation time and accuracy which is comparable to the effect shown by SS, although relatively more severe. This is accompanied by a milder morphemic dyslexia which is indexed by a high error rate and slow responses when reading lower frequency words. It is possible that the morphemic effect is a secondary consequence of the phonological impairment. However, this cannot be sustained as a general principle of causation since AD, SS and the competent readers JK and JS demonstrated that efficient functioning within the morphemic routes was compatible with an impairment of route 'g'.

TABLE 6.27   *Summary of cognitive description of reading functions of subject FM*

Function	Status	Comment
'm' → phonology	Mildly impaired	Large frequency effect. Grapheme-phoneme support for low frequency words. A few derivational errors. Serial processing
'g' → phonology	Impaired accuracy and latency	Difficulty with complex vowels. Lexical support. Slow serial processing
'm' → semantics	Effect on decision time	Large frequency effect. Typicality and relatedness effects. Serial processing in semantic decision task
Visual processor	Efficient matching Impaired format resolution	Slow serial processing. Slow format resolution

FM also gave evidence of a visual processor impairment. Her reading tended to be somewhat slow and serial and was vulnerable to disruption by format distortion. This pattern is different from that shown by RO and MF, particularly with regard to the presence of serial word reading and the absence of an effect on the general level of efficiency in the matching tasks.

Case II.2   David P (born July 1965)

1   Psycho-educational background

David's parents requested an assessment in 1978 stating that he had earlier produced mirror writing, that he still confused 'b' and 'd', that he had spelling difficulties and that he was left-handed for writing but right-handed for sports. An assessment using an abbreviated WISC showed his intelligence to be somewhat above average (full scale IQ = 109) although there was a retardation of about three years on the Daniels and Diack spelling test and on the accuracy and comprehension scales of the Neale Analysis of Reading. The psychologist noted a low score on the digit span sub-test and diagnosed a 'short-term memory impairment' and a specific disability in reading. The parents were advised to request an assessment by the child guidance service and to seek to arrange for remedial help in reading and spelling.

A further assessment was carried out in 1984 at the end of the research project. Administration of the WAIS gave the scaled scores listed in Table 6.28. These confirm the earlier testing, showing similar above average scores for the Verbal and Performance scales. The table also gives details of assessment of reading and spelling carried out in 1978 and 1984. These indicate progression towards a good level of competence in reading and slightly poorer performance in spelling. The psychologist commented that the reading errors were principally visual confusions and that this indication of inattention to detail was consistent with the relatively poor score on the picture completion tests of the WAIS. Reading comprehension was at ceiling for the tests. Spelling errors involved order confusions, b/d reversals, letter omissions, addition of an inappropriate final -e, and phonetically accurate attempts. Free writing was satisfactory with respect to quantity, legibility, expression and punctuation, although spelling was weak.

TABLE 6.28 *Results of administration of tests to subject DP (a) in 1978 when subject's CA was 13-1 years and (b) in 1984 when subject's CA was 19-4 years*

	IQ scores		Reading scores		Spelling scores
	WISC-R		Neale Analysis		Daniels and Diack
	full	109	rate	13-0 years	10-2 years
	verbal	104	accuracy	9-1 years	
a	performance	114	comprehension	10-10 years	
	WAIS		Schonell (test A)		Schonell (test A)
	Verbal IQ	113		13-0 years	12-5 years
	Information	10	Daniels and Diack		
	Similarities	12		(test 12)	
	Arithmetic	10		14+	
	Comprehension	15	Schonell (R4 test)		
b	Vocabulary	13		at ceiling	
	Digit span	11			
	Performance IQ	116			
	Picture completion	9			
	Picture arrangement	17			
	Block design	13			
	Object assembly	11			
	Digit symbol	12			

Other tests were generally negative. The score on the Bangor Dyslexia test was not significant. There was no evidence of impairment on the Graham Kendall Memory for Designs tests. The score on the Lindamood

Auditory Conceptualisation test was 88/100. This is considered predictive of difficulties at the upper primary level but the psychologist did not consider that the errors made by DP were suggestive of any serious difficulty in auditory processing.

No relevant information regarding DP's birth and early developmental history was available. Learning difficulties appear to have been suspected from early in primary school on account of the mirror writing and persistent b/d confusion. Remedial help was provided throughout his time at school. He was successful in his 'O' Grade examinations, obtaining passes in nine subjects. After leaving school he attended a college and sat some Higher Grade examinations, but without success. He then entered his father's business, though he states that he would like a more physical career, perhaps in the forces. His hobbies are sport in all forms, keeping fit, and music (drumming). He reads about three books per year for pleasure.

2 Experimental data

The experimental analysis of DP's reading functions confirmed the presence of only a mild degree of impairment. Table 6.29 summarises reaction time data for vocalisation of high frequency words, low frequency words and non-words. The reaction time distributions are displayed in Figure 6.5.

TABLE 6.29 *Vocal reaction times (ms) and error rates for reading high frequency words, low frequency words and non-words by DP*

| | High frequency words | | | Low frequency words | | | Non-words | | |
	Overall	Intercept	Slope	Overall	Intercept	Slope	Overall	Intercept	Slope
$\bar{X}$	1132	798	70[1]	1455	1257	42	1795	220	328[1]
sd	398			634			1007		
Error %	2.4			5.6			12.29		

[1] Linear trend significant at $p < 0.05$ or better by F-test
  Frequency effect: $t(279) = 5.212$, $p < 0.001$. $\chi^2(1) = 2.025$
  Lexicality effect (HF v NW): $t(368) = 7.903$, $p < 0.001$. $\chi^2(1) = 12.731$, $p < 0.001$
    (LF v NW): $t(323) = 3.3$, $p < 0.001$. $\chi^2(1) = 4.071$, $p < 0.05$

Word reading was very accurate. The reaction time distributions for both high and low frequency items were well formed but were more dispersed and somewhat higher in mean than the results for the competent readers. This slight overall slowness could be indicative of a morphemic effect, albeit one which was quite mild in its impact. There were no effects, on either accuracy or reaction time, of the content-function variable or of concrete versus abstract meaning. However, spelling-to-sound irregularity slowed responses to both high and low frequency words by more than 300 ms ($p < 0.01$) and raised the error rate for low frequency words from 0 to 17.86 per cent ($p < 0.05$). This suggests that DP's word reading was not

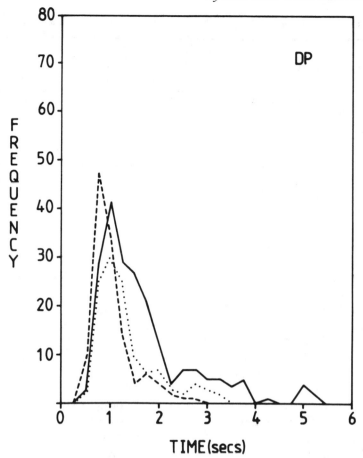

FIGURE 6.5   *Reaction time distributions for responses to high frequency words (– – –), low frequency words (. . .) and non-words (———) by DP*

supported by semantic processes but that there was some involvement of grapheme-phoneme translation.

The non-word distribution contained a preponderance of times < 2000 ms together with an appreciable tail of slower responses. Non-word reading was quite accurate (12 per cent error rate) and the differences between non-words and low frequency words were not unduly large. Only a mild phonological impairment is indicated. Homophony had no detectable effect on either the accuracy or the latency of non-word reading.

DP's reading errors included some phonetic regularisations (sew → 'sue', ski → 'sky', comb → 'com', aisle → 'isel'). There were also visual confusions between words (through → 'thought', winter → 'winner') and various errors involving the displacement, omission and insertion of sounds. Some of these involved lexicalised responses to non-words (e.g. dettis →

TABLE 6.30   *Reaction time (ms) and error data for lexical and semantic decisions by DP*

	HF words	LF words	Lexical decisions Legal non-words	Illegal non-words	All
$\bar{\text{X}}$	865	1290^2	2133	1095^2	1193
sd	301	746	1184	467	744
Error %	2.63	9.09	25^3	0	6.67
Rate (ms/letter)		124^1	126	33	114

[1] Significant linear trend
[2] Significant effect on reaction time
[3] Significant effect on error rate

'dentist', scrue → 'secure'). Others appeared to be simple errors of translation (plit → 'pilt', spooch → 'spoolch', litizun → 'litzun'). The structural analysis of the errors gave an average similarity score of 67 per cent, with translation least accurate for complex consonants. A few responses to non-words showed a use of V+C correspondences (e.g. halk → 'hawk'), but these accounted for no more than 8 per cent of responses on the list designed to test for this effect. The availability of an effective translation channel operating on simple correspondences without reference to stored vocabulary seems to be indicated.

Table 6.30 contains the results for the lexical and semantic decision tasks. Semantic decisions were accurately made and showed no obvious delay of reaction time. Lexical decisions were also efficient, though subject to a large frequency effect (400 ms) and to a marked elevation of the reaction time for rejection of legal non-words (over 2000 ms). If it can be assumed that this effect depends on an involvement of the mildly impaired translation channel, then it is probably reasonable to conclude that the morphemic route to semantics was efficient.

Results from the visual matching experiments, summarised in Table 6.31, are also suggestive of efficient functioning. Performance on the identity matching tasks was well within the competent reader range and reaction time was unaffected by variations in display size. The three array matching experiments also showed reaction time and error levels which were well within the normal range. There was evidence of left-to-right processing but the rate was no slower than that found for competent readers who processed the arrays serially. Orthographic legality did not affect accuracy or reaction time.

The effects of variations in word length have been included in Tables 6.29 and 6.30. There was a slow processing rate of 328 ms/letter in non-word reading. This is probably an aspect of DP's mild phonological impairment and suggests that the relatively wide dispersion of his non-word

| Typical positives | Semantic decisions | | | All |
	Atypical positives	Related negatives	Unrelated negatives	
1300	1369	1756	1691	1534
561	472	676	548	604
3.45	17.24	10	3.33	8.47
				126[1]

TABLE 6.31 *Reaction time (ms) and error rates for visual matching tasks by DP*

Experiment	Identity matching	Overall	Rate (ms/letter)		Array matching	Overall	Position of difference (ms/position)
1	$\bar{X}$	735	6	$\bar{X}$		1099	165[1]
	sd	256		sd		427	
	Error %	1.67		Error %		4	
2	$\bar{X}$	630	7	$\bar{X}$		1497	258[1]
	sd	199		sd		667	
	Error %	3.7		Error %		7.5	
3	$\bar{X}$	627	−5	$\bar{X}$		1557	151[1]
	sd	194		sd		641	
	Error %	215		Error %		6.25	

[1] Linear trend significant at $p<0.05$ or better by F-test

reaction time distribution (see Figure 6.5) was attributable in part to reliance on a slow serial process when attempting to read these items. Word reading and semantic decision making gave some evidence of serial processing although the rates were within or at the upper limit of the normal range. There was a large effect of length on positive lexical decisions. Removal of one outlying reaction time reduced this to 124 ms/letter, but this value remains substantial and reflected a significant linear trend. Overall, therefore, DP's reading contains evidence of serial processing although the effect is not a major one.

Table 6.32 contains a summary of the format distortion data. High frequency word reading, semantic decisions and lexical decisions all gave evidence of processing rates which were slow but which lay at the upper limit of the normal range. The exceptions to this generalisation were the rates of 340 ms/letter and of 500 ms/letter found for low frequency words and for non-words.

TABLE 6.32   *Reaction times (ms) and error rates for reading normal and distorted words or non-words by DP*

		Vocalisation tasks		Decision tasks	
		Words	Non-words	Semantic	Lexical
Normal	X̄	1024	1829	1213	1299
	sd	379	975	576	927
	Error %	3.33	26.67	8.33	5
	Rate	115^1	273^1	123^1	139
Zigzag	X̄	1210	2381	1424^2	1358
	sd	531	1349	354	538
	Error %	0	16.67	0^3	5
	Rate	156^1	480^1	13	155^1
Vertical	X̄	1547^2	2351	1747^2	1599^2
	sd	710	1150	725	792
	Error %	6.67	23.33	8.51	6.67
	Rate	300^1	500^1	249^1	186^1

[1] Significant linear trend
[2] Format effect on reaction time
[3] Format effect on accuracy

3   Conclusions

DP's results suggest that he may be an 'ex-dyslexic', who encountered difficulties during childhood which were quite well resolved by the end of his school career. His Level I (competence) description indicated above average intelligence combined with competent reading and some residual spelling difficulties. There were no clear indications of any accompanying deficits.

The Level II (cognitive) analysis suggested the presence of a mild phonological dyslexia, principally affecting translation time, combined with efficient functioning in the other domains. Hints of a more general impairment were given by DP's relatively high reading reaction times and a tendency towards slightly slow serial processing, especially when resolving distortions.

A statement of DP's cognitive description, expressed in the terms of the four domains of the processing model, appears in Table 6.33. In summary, DP might be classed as a 'normal reader' whose processing system retains some dyslexic traces.

TABLE 6.33   *Summary of cognitive description of reading functions of subject DP*

Function	Status	Comment
'm' → phonology	Very mild effect	Large frequency effect. Grapheme-phoneme support
'g' → phonology	Mild effect	Simple correspondences. Slow serial processing
'm' → semantics	Efficient	Frequency effect. Serial processing in lexical decision task
Visual processor	Efficient	Slow distortion resolution for non-words

Case II.3   Claire E (born October 1968)

1   Psycho-educational background

Claire E was born by forceps delivery at full term on account of foetal distress and was kept under special observation during the first 24 hours of life. Early developmental milestones were normal. Her parents, a college lecturer and primary teacher, suspected learning difficulties when they observed that, although she seemed to be a competent reader, she was experiencing persistent difficulties in spelling and writing. Following an assessment by the Tayside Dyslexia Association in 1980 individual tuition was arranged and was maintained over a two year period. Claire was granted a spelling concession for her 'O' Grades and passed six subjects. In 1985 she was preparing to sit four subjects at the Higher Grade but was uncertain what she wished to do after leaving school. She enjoys music and reads four or five books a month for pleasure. It was reported that her father had experienced spelling difficulties.

CE was assessed by administration of an abbreviated WISC in 1980. The scaled scores appear in Table 6.34 and can be seen to indicate an above average intelligence level (full scale IQ = 112). The results of retesting with the full WISC in 1984 also appear in Table 6.34. These scores are at an average level and reveal no surprising features. The psychologist considered that Claire was poorly motivated during the testing and that this might explain the fall in her scores.

Claire's reading was assessed at various points between 1980 and 1984. The results of these tests have been summarised in Table 6.35. The scores tend to confirm the absence of a severe difficulty in reading. Results from spelling tests, also shown in the table, are indicative of a special problem in this area.

In 1980 an administration of the Wepman Auditory Discrimination test revealed a good level of accuracy with very slow responding. On this account, the psychologist concluded that her spelling difficulties might be of

TABLE 6.34   *Results of administration of the WISC to subject CE (a) in 1980 when subject's CA was 11-8 years and (b) in 1984 when subject's CA was 16-2 years*

	a				b		
Verbal tests		Performance tests		Verbal tests		Performance tests	
Similarities	13	Block design	10	Similarities	8	Block design	10
Arithmetic	9	Object assembly	12	Arithmetic	10	Object assembly	9
Vocabulary	12	Mazes	13	Vocabulary	11	Picture completion	11
Digit span	12			Digit span	13	Picture arrangement	9
				Information	9	Coding	10
				Comprehension	9		
Verbal IQ	114	Performance IQ	106	Verbal IQ	96	Performance IQ	98

TABLE 6.35   *Results of administration of reading and spelling tests to subject CE (a) in 1980 when subject's CA was 11-8 years, (b) in 1982 when subject's CA was 13-9 years and (c) in 1984 when subject's CA was 16-2 years*

		Reading scores		Spelling scores
a	Neale Analysis			Daniels and Diack
	rate		11-2 yrs	8-5 yrs
	accuracy		10-2 yrs	
	comprehension		12-4 yrs	
b	Daniels and Diack		12-6 yrs	Daniels and Diack
				9-2 yrs
c	Schonell (test A)		13-0 yrs	Schonell (test A)
				11-6 yrs
	Daniels and Diack (test 12)		13-7 yrs	
	Schonell (R4 test)		12-6 yrs	

an 'auditory dyslexic type'. The Lindamood test of Auditory Conceptualisation was administered in 1984. Her score of 81/100 was considered predictive of reading and spelling difficulties at the middle primary level.

Orthoptics testing in 1984 revealed no visual anomalies and the establishment of a fixed right reference eye. Claire was also right-handed and footed. The Graham Kendall Memory for Designs test gave a difference score of 2 which was said to be indicative of 'borderline neurological dysfunction', and to suggest that a general impairment of shape memory might be related to her spelling problems.

On the Bangor Dyslexia test Claire had difficulty with left-right discrimination, compass point directions and repetition of polysyllables. Her mother reported that she had had difficulty in learning to read the clock and that she showed an above average tendency towards the production of Spoonerisms.

2   Experimental data

CE's results for reading high frequency words, low frequency words and non-words appear in Table 6.36. The distributions of reaction times appear in Figure 6.6. Word reading was accurate and the distributions contained a preponderance of times <2000 ms. Nonetheless, the overall level of the reaction time was elevated relative to the data from the competent reader sample and the distributions included some slow and outlying responses. The word frequency effect, at 400 ms, was also large. These features are suggestive of a mild morphemic dyslexia.

TABLE 6.36   *Vocal reaction times (ms) and error rates for reading high frequency words, low frequency words and non-words by CE*

	High frequency words			Low frequency words			Non-words		
	Overall	Intercept	Slope	Overall	Intercept	Slope	Overall	Intercept	Slope
X̄	1194	870	68[1]	1594	276	282[1]	2440	387	427[1]
sd	520			1059			1707		
Error %	2.98		.	9.52			18.22		

[1] Linear trend significant at p<0.05 or better by F-test
  Frequency effect: $t(275) = 4.141$, $p<0.001$. $\chi^2(1) = 5.666$, $p<0.02$
  Lexicality effect (HF v NW):$t(354) = 8.946$, $p<0.001$. $\chi^2(1) = 21.783$, $p<0.001$
      (LF v NW):$t(305) = 4.759$, $p<0.001$. $\chi^2(1) = 4.821$, $p<0.05$

Non-word reading was subject to a relatively high error rate (18 per cent). The reaction time level was high at over 2400 ms and the distribution was widely dispersed and included numerous slow responses. The results are indicative of a phonological impairment.

CE's word reading was not affected by the semantic/syntactic variables of form class and concreteness. However, spelling-to-sound irregularity affected low frequency word reading, increasing error rate from 0 to 25 per cent (p<0.05) and raising the reaction time by 500 ms (p<0.01). This suggests that grapheme-phoneme translation was used to support word retrieval. The occurrence of a few regularisation errors (come → 'comb', corps → 'corpse', ski → 'sky', aisle → 'asel', ache → 'arch') is consistent with this conclusion. There were also effects of non-word homophony, which reduced errors in non-word reading from 20 to 5 per cent, and reaction time from 3400 ms to 2400 ms (p<0.01). This suggests that the translation process was sometimes supported by matching against items in the vocabulary store.

An analysis of CE's errors in the vocalisation tasks did not reveal any unusual features. There was an even distribution of word and non-word

TABLE 6.37   *Reaction times (ms) and error data for lexical and semantic decisions by CE*

		HF words	LF words	Lexical decisions Legal non-words	Illegal non-words	All
	X	1167	1514^2	2669^2	2116	1750
	sd	481	564	1090	872	910
Error	%	7.89	9.09	35^2	12.2	14.05
Rate (ms/letter)		129		266	42	105

[1] Significant linear trend
[2] Significant effect on reaction time
[3] Significant effect on error rate

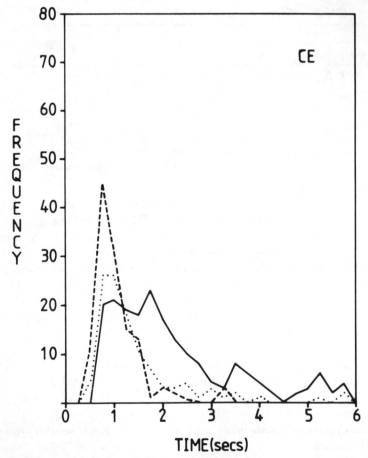

FIGURE 6.6   *Reaction time distributions for responses to high frequency words (– – –), low frequency words (. . .) and non-words (———) by CE*

Typical positives	Atypical positives	Semantic decisions Related negatives	Unrelated negatives	All
1950	2193	2870	2397	2321
864	877	1286	734	987
6.67	6.9	27.59^3	0	10.17
				195^1

responses. Responses were structurally similar to their targets (average similarity score = 73 per cent) and involved numerous vowel misreadings plus some consonant confusions. The cluster match scores ranged from 82 per cent correct for simple consonants down to 23 per cent correct for complex vowels. Use of major correspondences in non-word reading was infrequent (about 10 per cent of responses in the experiment varying lexical environment).

CE's results from the decision experiments appear in Table 6.37. The reaction time for semantic decisions was high at over 2300 ms, and the distribution was dispersed with a tail of slow responses. Lexical decisions also gave evidence of slowness of response, particularly affecting both legal and illegal non-words. There was a high error rate (35 per cent) on the legal non-words. The frequency effect on positive RT was over 300 ms. The slowness of response in these tasks is suggestive of a mild impairment of the morphemic route to semantics.

The results from the matching experiments have been summarised in Table 6.38. These data are clearly indicative of a marked visual processor impairment which affects the speed, though not the accuracy, of visual comparisons. Reaction times in identity matching were dispersed and the mean levels lay well above the range for the competent readers. The reaction time for array matching was extremely high (greater than 3500 ms). There was no significant effect of the legality of the letter arrays. The data were very variable and the position of difference functions were generally not significant on the linear trend test. This suggests that CE was not operating a systematically programmed left-to-right processing strategy.

The second indicator of visual processor functions to be considered is the effect of word length on the reaction time. The relevant data appear in Tables 6.36 and 6.37. The rates for lexical decisions appear quite high, but the linear trends were not significant. Semantic decisions were also made with a rate somewhat above the normal range. However, the figure in the

TABLE 6.38   *Reaction times (ms) and error rates for visual matching tasks by CE*

| Experiment | | Identity matching | | | Array matching | |
		Overall	Rate (ms/letter)		Overall	Position of difference (ms/position)
1	$\bar{X}$	1648	38	$\bar{X}$	3597	289
	sd	890		sd	2838	
	Error %	0		Error %	5	
2	$\bar{X}$	2179	58	$\bar{X}$	4711	464
	sd	1270		sd	4149	
	Error %	1.23		Error %	9.24	
3	$\bar{X}$	1359	−49[1]	$\bar{X}$	4545	435[1]
	sd	888		sd	2881	
	Error %	0		Error %	3.13	

[1] Linear trend significant at $p<0.05$ or better by F-test

table is based on a distribution which includes a number of outliers. If these are removed by setting a cut-off at the boundary of the main distribution (3000 ms) the estimate of the processing rate falls to 72 ms/letter. The linear trend was significant, but the obtained value is well within the range for the normal readers. Thus, the data do not give evidence of serial processing in tasks involving semantic access.

The vocalisation experiments gave slightly stronger evidence of serial processing. The rate for high frequency words (68 ms/letter) was somewhat above the range for the competent readers although relatively fast. Low frequency words were read at a much slower rate. However, a reanalysis with outliers >3000 ms removed reduced the rate to 97 ms/letter. These analyses suggest that there was a serial element in the process of accessing phonology via route 'm' but that the processing rate was quite fast. Non-word reading, by contrast, was achieved with the very slow rate of 427 ms/letter. This suggests that part of the reason for the wide dispersion of CE's non-word distribution was a dependence on slow serial handling during translation.

These results are in many respects similar to those obtained from subjects RO and MF. The interpretation of their data in terms of an impairment of the analytic function of the visual processor was based on the coincidence of slow matching performance, slow serial processing in non-word reading, and slow serial processing in tasks requiring the resolution of format distortions. The format distortion results, summarised in Table 6.39, indicate that CE exhibited a very similar pattern. Her processing rates for resolution of the vertical distortions were well in excess of the upper limit for the normal range in both the vocalisation and the decision tasks.

TABLE 6.39   *Reaction times (ms) and error rates for reading normal and distorted words or non-words by CE*

		Vocalisation tasks		Decision tasks	
		Words	Non-words	Semantic	Lexical
Normal	$\bar{X}$	1414	2068	2876	3129
	sd	431	970	1535	1651
Error %		0	13.33	2.13	8.33
	Rate	162[1]	386[1]	15	252
Zigzag	$\bar{X}$	1993[2]	4497[2]	3041	3677
	sd	800	3494	1178	1835
Error %		6.67	20	6.38	3.33
	Rate	250[1]	1202[1]	145	124
Vertical	$\bar{X}$	3174[2]	3318[2]	3662[2]	3819[2]
	sd	2264	1854	1774	1743
Error %		10	16.67	6.25	6.67
	Rate	931[1]	752[1]	586[1]	393[1]

[1] Significant linear trend
[2] Format effect on reaction time
[3] Format effect on accuracy

3   Conclusions

CE's Level I (cognitive) description defines her as a girl of average ability whose dyslexic problems are concerned with spelling rather than with reading. There are indications of accompanying impairments affecting audition and language and visual memory.

The Level II (cognitive) description is indicative of a marked visual processor impairment accompanied by mild effects on the morphemic channels and a relatively stronger effect on the grapheme-phoneme translation channel. Table 6.40 contains a summary of CE's cognitive description.

TABLE 6.40   *Summary of cognitive description of reading functions of subject CE*

Function	Status	Comment
'm' → phonology	Mildly impaired	Large frequency effect. Grapheme-phoneme support for low frequency words
'g' → phonology	Impaired	Lexical support. Difficulty with complex vowels. Slow serial processing
'm' → semantics	Mildly impaired	Frequency effect
Visual processor	Impaired	Slow identity matching. Very slow array matching. Slow format resolution

CE's visual processor impairment appears to be similar to that shown by RO and MF. The processor had difficulty in operating analytically in order to make visual comparisons, to resolve distortions or to segment non-words. She differs from RO and MF in showing a larger effect on translation time and a tendency to refer output from the translator to the speech production lexicon. In addition, she gives evidence of mild morphemic impairments. There is at present no basis for deciding whether these effects are aspects of a generalised inefficiency, analogous to that shown by the competent reader, LL, or whether the morphemic effects are consequent on the primary visual processor impairment.

Case II.4   David T (born May 1964)

1   Psycho-educational background

David T's mother reported that she had been aware of problems from an early stage of his schooling. One-to-one tuition was arranged and carried on over a period of years until a pass in 'O' Grade English was achieved. At the start of the project in 1981 David was in his sixth year at secondary school and was hoping to proceed to a degree course in engineering. He was studying Mathematics and Engineering Science at CSYS level and Technical Drawing at the Higher Grade. In his fourth year at school he had obtained 'O' Grade passes in Technical Drawing, Engineering Science, Physics, Chemistry, Mathematics, Geography and Arithmetic, but had failed English. He succeeded in passing English the following year, and also obtained Higher Grade passes in Physics, Engineering Science, Mathematics and Chemistry. This academic performance is suggestive of a high level of ability in the numerical/spatial fields. An administration of the Similarities, Vocabulary, Digit span, Block design and Object assembly sub-tests of the WISC-R in 1982 gave scaled scores of 17 for the two performance tests, and of 13 and 11 for the two verbal tests. Digit span was depressed with a score of 6. The scores suggest a markedly superior performance IQ combined with average verbal intelligence and a possible deficit in verbal short-term memory. An assessment of reading and spelling carried out in the same year with the Schonell Graded Word tests gave a reading age of 12-6+ years and a spelling age of 12-1 years.

2   Experimental data

DT's results for reading high and low frequency words and non-words have been summarised in Table 6.41. The reaction time distributions are displayed in Figure 6.7. The data are suggestive of a phonological dyslexia, since non-word reading was carried out with an elevated reaction time (2280 ms) and dispersed distribution, and a relatively large difference between non-words and low frequency words (736 ms). However, words were also read with a reaction time somewhat above the level of the competent readers and the distributions were well formed but quite widely dispersed. This slowness of response to familiar words appears indicative of a mild morphemic dyslexia.

TABLE 6.41 *Vocal reaction times (ms) and error rates for reading high frequency words, low frequency words and non-words by DT*

| | High frequency words | | | Low frequency words | | | Non-words | | |
	Overall	Intercept	Slope	Overall	Intercept	Slope	Overall	Intercept	Slope
$\bar{X}$	1383	843	113[1]	1543	1116	91[1]	2279	830	299[1]
sd	493			553			1012		
Error %	1.79			7.14			14.83		

[1] Linear trend significant at $p<0.05$ or better by F-test
Frequency effect: $t(280) = 2.541$, $p<0.01$. $\chi^2(1) = 5.278$, $p<0.05$
Lexicality effect (HF v NW): $t(364) = 10.368$, $p<0.001$. $\chi^2(1) = 19.598$, $p<0.001$
(LF v NW): $t(316) = 7.234$, $p<0.001$. $\chi^2(1) = 4.547$, $p<0.05$

The analysis of psycholinguistic effects on word reading gave no evidence of an impact of concrete versus abstract meaning although function words were read 190 ms slower than high frequency content words ($p<0.05$). A deficit in function word reading has sometimes been noted in accounts of cases of acquired phonological dyslexia (Patterson, 1982). Spelling-to-sound irregularity had no effect on high frequency word reading but increased reaction time by 275 ms for low frequency words and raised the error rate from 3.57 per cent to 25 per cent ($p<0.05$). These effects suggest that, despite the phonological dyslexia, DT made use of grapheme-phoneme translation when attempting to retrieve responses to lower frequency words. The occurrence of some regularisation errors (sew → 'sue', corps → 'corpse', heir → 'hair', aisle → 'isel', comb with the 'b' pronounced) supports this conclusion.

The results of the non-word reading experiment showed that homophony produced a 457 ms effect on reaction time ($p<0.025$), but no effect on accuracy. This suggests that grapheme-phoneme translation was occasionally supported by reference to the vocabulary store in the phonological processor.

Given this evidence for non-lexical processing during word reading, and for lexicalisation of responses to non-words, it would be anticipated that DT's error set should include both words and neologisms. Table 6.42 gives the frequencies of word and non-word responses to word and non-word targets, together with the reaction time associated with each error type. Word and non-word responses occurred with approximately equal frequencies. There was a reaction time difference of 1800 ms between word → word errors, such as liberty → 'library', and non-word → non-

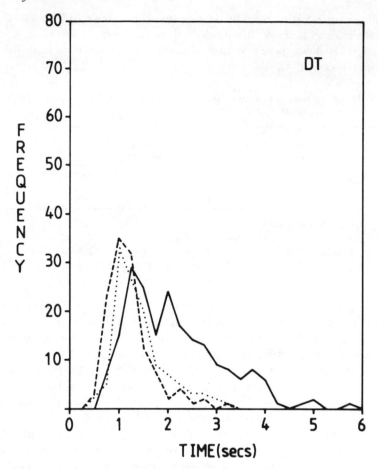

FIGURE 6.7   *Reaction time distributions for responses to high frequency words (– – –), low frequency words (. . .) and non-words (——) by DT*

word errors, such as slooch → 'slosh' (p<0.01). This effect is explicable on the assumption that word-word errors reflect confusions within the morphemic channel, whereas non-word → non-word errors derive from translation failures in the slower grapheme-phoneme channel. DT's error latencies also give evidence of lexicalisation of responses to non-words. Word responses to non-words, e.g. trast → 'trash', were made 1221 ms faster than non-word responses to non-words (p<0.01). It seems unlikely that these responses were produced by the same process as the word-word errors, since they had a significantly slower mean latency.

TABLE 6.42 *Error frequencies and reaction times (ms) classified by target and response lexicality for DT*

| | Word targets | | Non-word targets | |
	Words	Non-words	Words	Non-words
X̄	1592	2744	2173	3394
sd	723	1184	577	1765
N	9	3	16	19

DT's results from the decision tasks are summarised in Table 6.43. In general, these do not give evidence of an impairment of the morphemic route to semantics. Semantic decisions were very accurate, and the reaction time, although high (1539 ms), was within the competent reader range. Neither typicality nor relatedness exerted significant effects. Lexical decisions were made with a fast reaction time and about 10 per cent of errors, mainly failures to reject legal non-words. There was an effect of frequency on positive reaction time and a large effect of legality on negative RT and error rate.

The results from the visual matching tasks appear in Table 6.44. The data give no indication of a visual processor impairment. Both identity judgments and array comparisons were made with reaction times and error rates which were well within the normal range. There were no strong indications of serial processing and no effects of orthographic legality.

The effects of word length have been summarised in Tables 6.41 and 6.43. Processing rates in the lexical and semantic decision tasks were fast and statistically negligible. The rate for vocal responses to words, on the other hand, was about 100 ms/letter. This trend was significant and was not modified when four outlying reaction times >3000 ms were removed. The rate for non-word reading was somewhat slower, at nearly 300 ms/letter. These results suggest a distinction between the two morphemic routes, with the route to phonology being more dependent on serial processing than the route to semantics.

The results for the format distortion experiments have been summarised in Table 6.45. In two instances (word reading and semantic decisions) distortion produced effects which were within though close to the limit of the competent reader range. The effects on lexical decisions and non-word reading were somewhat greater. These data are equivocal with regard to the effects of distortion on DT's reading. However, the only really large effects were on non-word reading, which was already a slow serial process for DT. It may be reasonable to conclude, therefore, that DT does not show the major and consistent effects of distortion which were characteristic of subjects RO, MF and CE.

TABLE 6.43   *Reaction time (ms) and error data for lexical and semantic decisions by DT*

	HF words	LF words	Lexical decisions Legal non-words	Illegal non-words	All
X̄	950	1099^2	1321^2	821	962
sd	296	344	325	194	314
Error %	0	4.55	55^3	0	10
Rate (ms/letter)		4	38	−48	−10

[1] Significant linear trend
[2] Significant effect on reaction time
[3] Significant effect on error rate

TABLE 6.44   *Reaction times (ms) and error rates for visual matching tasks*

Experiment		Identity matching Overall	Rate (ms/letter)		Array matching Overall	Position of difference (ms/position)
1	X̄	851	11	X̄	1299	53
	sd	302		sd	507	
	Error %	0.83		Error %	1	
2	X̄	843	22^1	X̄	1472	102
	sd	305		sd	619	
	Error %	0		Error %	5	
3	X̄	981	2	X̄	1344	−18
	sd	412		sd	611	
	Error %	0.83		Error %	2.5	

[1] Linear trend significant at p<0.05 or better by F-test

3   Conclusions

DT's Level I description defines him as an individual of superior non-verbal intelligence who encountered, but successfully overcame, some dyslexic difficulties during his time at school.

The Level II description is indicative of a relatively mild phonological dyslexia combined with a small morphemic effect on the route for accessing phonology. Table 6.46 contains a summary of the conclusions regarding each of the four processing domains. The description suggests that DT suffers a residual phonological dyslexia, principally affecting translation time. He has an operational translator which is used in conjunction with the morphemic channel. The observation that word length exerted much

| Typical positives | Semantic decisions | | | All |
	Atypical positives	Related negatives	Unrelated negatives	
1180	1357	1846	1737	1539
396	660	625	756	682
0	10.34	3.33	0	3.42
				31

TABLE 6.45   *Reaction times (ms) and error rates for reading normal and distorted words or non-words by DT*

| | | Vocalisation tasks | | Decision tasks | |
		Words	Non-words	Semantic	Lexical
Normal	$\bar{X}$	1323	3055	1382	1370
	sd	463	1656	585	752
Error %		0	3.33	2.08	6.67
	Rate	53	115	41	−51
Zigzag	$\bar{X}$	1558	3931[2]	1610[2]	1826[2]
	sd	751	1657	517	1109
Error %		16.67[3]	10	2.08	11.67
	Rate	202[1]	686[1]	23	86
Vertical	$\bar{X}$	1886[2]	3274	1790[2]	2015[2]
	sd	809	1610	774	1154
Error %		6.67	10	4.26	13.33
	Rate	241[1]	395[1]	236	220[1]

[1] Significant linear trend
[2] Format effect on reaction time
[3] Format effect on accuracy

greater effects on vocalisation than on lexical or semantic decisions suggests that the two morphemic routes relied on different forms of visual processing. It may be that grapheme-phoneme translation, involving segmentation and serial processing, was typically required for route 'm' to phonology.

Conclusions: Series II

The second series of cases confirmed the conclusion that a variety of dyslexic patterns can be found. Subjects DP and DT appeared to be cases

TABLE 6.46   *Summary of cognitive description of reading functions of subject DT*

Function	Status	Comment
'm' < phonology	Very mild effect	Frequency effect. Function word effect. Grapheme-phoneme support for low frequency words. Regularisation errors. Serial processing
'g' < phonology	Mild effect on translation time	Lexicalisation. Slow serial processing
'm' < semantics	Efficient	Frequency effect
Visual processor	Efficient	Slow format resolution for non-words

of recovery from dyslexia who gave evidence of a diffusely distributed but mild slowing of processing speed. Subject CE provided further evidence of an impairment of visual processor functions of the kind found for RO and MF in Series I, although she differed from the two older subjects in displaying larger accompanying effects on the grapheme-phoneme and morphemic routes. Subject FM also showed a variety of impairments, but the main feature seemed to be a phonological dyslexia combined with some morphemic effects.

6.5   Conclusions

This chapter has presented the results of cognitive analyses of 8 dyslexic subjects whose reading was relatively unimpaired according to Level I criteria. Nonetheless, the subjects all exhibited some localised information processing inefficiencies.

It seems clear that the pattern of impairments does not remain constant as the successive cases are reviewed. Therefore, the proposal that developmental dyslexia might reasonably be treated as a homogeneous category may be rejected with respect to this sample. The results reported in Chapter 5 suggest that the proposal may also be rejected for the sample of younger competent readers.

A preliminary conclusion is that 'developmental dyslexia' will prove to be a heterogeneous category when subjected to a detailed cognitive analysis of individual cases. It is probably too early to comment on the relative merits of the heterogeneity and sub-type proposals. However, the results do not encourage the view that configurations featuring a distinctive impairment and associated pattern of effects can be identified. The data more obviously favour the conclusion that the systems postulated in the model may be affected singly or in combination, thus generating a large variety of configurations.

For these reasons it may be best to stand by the earlier conclusion that dyslexia can most profitably be discussed by analysing impairments of specific systems or pathways.

Impairment of route 'g' to phonology

The results confirm the findings from the competent reader sample by demonstrating that route 'g' may be impaired with respect to accuracy, or translation time, or both. Subject AD showed an accuracy effect, subject DT a processing time effect, and subjects SS and FM effects on accuracy and time. The results also support the conclusion that a phonological impairment of this type does not necessarily compromise the operation of the morphemic routes.

In the approach to the analysis of 'acquired dyslexia' initiated by Marshall and Newcombe (1973) it has been usual to think in terms of an impairment of one route forcing a reliance on a less impaired process. Thus, phonological dyslexia should be characterised by an inability to use grapheme-phoneme translation and a tendency to rely on semantic processing. The discussions of strategic options suggest that this form of compensation was not adopted by the subjects in the present series. AD, SS, FM and DT all gave evidence of the use of the grapheme-phoneme channel in word reading, whereas only SS and DT gave some indications of semantic effects. There was also no general tendency for non-word reading to be supported by reference to the lexicon (DT and, to a lesser extent, FM showed this effect but AD and SS did not).

Non-word reading appeared to be based primarily on primitive grapheme-phoneme correspondences. The errors were generally structurally similar to the targets and involved minor confusions over letter identities and positions, with the difficulties focusing on complex graphemic structures, especially the vowels. It was generally true that an impairment of translation time reflected a reliance on slow serial processing of non-words.

Visual processor impairments

Subjects RO, MF and CE were considered to give evidence of an impairment localised within the visual processor. These subjects presented a conjunction of effects in which the predominant features were: elevation of the RT in the identity matching and array matching experiments; slow processing rates in resolution of format distortions (especially the vertical distortion); and a tendency towards slow serial processing in non-word reading. This pattern has been interpreted as an impairment of the analytic mode of the visual processor. The results suggest that the impairment does not have necessary consequences for the operation of the morphemic routes but that it does slow down the rate of functioning of route 'g'.

The results from the other subjects gave weaker indications of visual processor effects. Subject AD was affected by graphemic complexity and shared with SS, FM, DP and DT a slight slowness in dealing with the distortions, particularly when reading non-words. It seems possible that there can be a 'downstream' effect from the phonological processor to the visual processor, such that limitations on translation speed affect visual processor operations and combine with the distortions to produce large disruptive effects. There was also evidence from the results of FM and DP of slow serial reading of words.

The effects of the orthographic legality were somewhat inconsistent. The Series I subjects all showed large legality effects in the array matching task and in the lexical decision experiments. These effects were taken to imply the availability of an orthographic model of spelling patterns within the processor. In Series II, the lexical decision effects were variable and there were no significant effects in the matching task.

Morphemic effects

Effects on the morphemic pathways were indexed by errors in word reading and lexical or semantic decisions, and by dispersal of the reaction time distributions. There was no evidence of such effects in the results of AD, SS and RO. Subjects DP and DT also appeared morphemically efficient, although the overall level of their reaction times was slightly elevated. MF and CE gave some evidence of morphemic effects in the form of slowness on the decision task and occasional indications of serial reading. These effects were more strongly present in the case of FM.

The morphemic effects appear to apply to both the phonological and the semantic routes and to be associated with a tendency towards slow serial reading, although this effect is not always equivalent across tasks.

7 Series III: morphemic dyslexia

7.1 Introduction

The previous chapter presented data for eight subjects in whom reading processes functioned relatively efficiently. The cases gave evidence of phonological effects on accuracy or translation time and of anomalies in the visual processor. These results confirmed that the establishment of efficient morphemic processes was possible in the context of an impaired visual processor or an impaired grapheme-phoneme translator. Some of the cases exhibited a more complex pattern in which visual or phonological effects were accompanied by evidence of a morphemic impairment. According to the arguments presented, these effects should be viewed as independent impairments and not as direct consequences of the visual or phonological disturbances.

In this chapter I will present the results of five further subjects who provide stronger evidence of morphemic effects. This group will be referred to as Series III and included four boys (AR, LA, SM and GS), all in the early stages of secondary schooling, and one girl, who was of below average general intelligence and who came from a disadvantaged social background. The subjects all gave evidence of a morphemic impairment in the form of delays or errors in word reading. They also showed some phonological effects. I included them in Series III only if the accompanying phonological effect was relatively mild. Subjects showing larger phonological effects will be considered in Chapter 8.

7.2 Series II case studies

The cases from Series III will be presented in an order which reflects their efficiency in reading high frequency words.

Case III.1   Alistair R (born April 1967)

1   Psycho-educational background

Alistair R was referred to the Tayside Dyslexia Association on the advice of his teacher. It was reported that his father had experienced some learning difficulties at school. He was found to be left-handed but right-eyed and right-footed. An intellectual assessment using an ˏ abbreviated WISC suggested an above average ability level (Verbal IQ = 109, Performance IQ = 121). His reading, assessed by the Neale test, was about 1-6 years behind his age. Spelling was quite severely impaired (spelling age = 6-7 years). In 1981, when he was aged 14 years, his scores on the Schonell tests were 11-10 years for reading and 10-4 years for spelling.

2   Experimental data

AR was tested by C. Porpodas when he was aged about 10 years (Seymour and Porpodas, 1980). His performance at that time appeared indicative of a combined morphemic and phonological dyslexia. The reaction time in non-word reading exceeded 300 ms with an error rate of over 21 per cent. His reading of words of regular spelling was also very slow and inaccurate. Lexical decisions involved numerous false rejections of words and were carried out with an elevated reaction time.

The results from the experiments administered in 1981 suggested that there had been considerable gains in efficiency in the intervening period. The data for reading high frequency words, low frequency words and non-words appear in Table 7.1. The reaction time distributions are displayed in Figure 7.1. Both the reaction time and the error levels were slightly above the range for the competent readers. The distributions were well formed but included a tail of slow responses. There was a large effect of word frequency (over 500 ms). These features appear indicative of a mild morphemic impairment.

TABLE 7.1   *Vocal reaction times (ms) and error rates for reading high frequency words, low frequency words and non-words by AR*

	High frequency words			Low frequency words			Non-words		
	Overall	Intercept	Slope	Overall	Intercept	Slope	Overall	Intercept	Slope
X̄	1117	476	133[1]	1642	1434	44	1653	729	191[1]
sd	540			2550			748		
Error %	5.36			11.11			13.14		

[1] Linear trend significant at p<0.05 or better by F-test
   Frequency effect: t(269) = 2.508, p<0.01. $\chi^2(1)$ = 3.306
   Lexicality effect (HF v NW):t(362) = 7.598, p<0.001. $\chi^2(1)$ = 6.656, p<0.01
            (LF v NW):t(315) = 0.057. $\chi^2(1)$ = 0.309

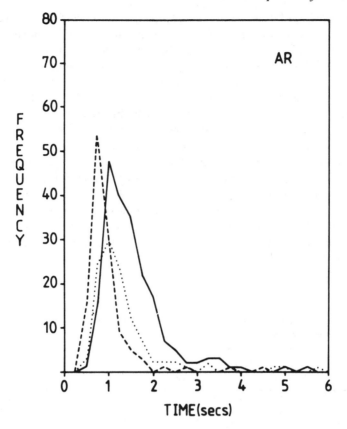

FIGURE 7.1   *Reaction time distributions for responses to high frequency words (– – –), low frequency words (. . .) and non-words (———) by AR*

The effect on non-word reading was relatively slight. The error rate, at 13 per cent, was within the range covered by the competent readers. There were some slow responses in the tail of the reaction time distribution but the overall latency was at about the level associated with a mild phonological effect. The differences between low frequency words and non-words (the lexicality effect) were not significant for either accuracy or reaction time.

These results suggest the presence of a balanced phonological and morphemic dyslexia both of which are mild in impact. Consistent with this dual effect, AR showed influences of both semantic and spelling-to-sound regularity variables on word reading. There was a delay of over 600 ms on the speed of reading abstract words (p<0.01). Irregularity raised error rate from 2 per cent to 20 per cent (p<0.01). These effects suggest that both semantic processing and grapheme-phoneme translation may have been used to assist word retrieval.

Non-word reading showed a small effect of vowel complexity on accuracy but no effects of homophony. In the experiment varying lexical environment, about 27 per cent of responses gave evidence of the use of higher order correspondences (e.g. galk → 'gawk', vull → /vɒl/, gind → /gaɪnd/, squant → /skwɒnt/). The initial /w/ rule was applied on all six occasions on which it was tested. These results suggest that the grapheme-phoneme channel, while operating independently of the speech production vocabulary, was nonetheless quite highly 'lexicalised' in the sense that it made use of correspondences above the grapheme-phoneme level.

A summary of AR's error distribution appears in Table 7.2. AR produced both word and non-word errors but response lexicality and target lexicality tended to covary ($p < 0.05$ by chi-square test). Error reaction times were faster for word than for non-word responses. The errors themselves were generally structurally close to their targets (average similarity score = 67 per cent), with translation errors tending to focus on the complex vowels.

TABLE 7.2   *Frequencies and latencies (ms) of word and non-word error responses to word and non-word targets by AR*

	Words		Non-words	
	Words	Non-words	Words	Non-words
$\overline{X}$	1838	8293	1381	3490
sd	1673	8352	306	4143
N	16	7	11	20

TABLE 7.3   *Reaction time (ms) and error data for lexical and semantic decisions by AR*

	Lexical decisions				
	HF words	LF words	Legal non-words	Illegal non-words	All
$\overline{X}$	1077	1222	1947[2]	1213	1259
sd	385	378	868	296	507
Error %	0	30[3]	30[3]	2.44	11.57
Rate	33		497[2]	59	113[1]
(ms/letter)					

[1] Significant linear trend
[2] Significant effect on reaction time
[3] Significant effect on error rate

The results from the decision experiments have been summarised in Table 7.3. The reaction time in semantic decisions was somewhat high (2000 ms) and the distribution included a substantial tail of slow responses. There were effects of both typicality and relatedness on error rate. Lexical decisions were made somewhat more efficiently, but there were error rates of about 30 per cent on both low frequency words and legal non-words. Legality had a large effect on both error rate and reaction time. The poor discrimination in lexical decisions combined with the slow responses in the semantic decision task are suggestive of a mild effect on route 'm' to semantics.

An analysis of the effects of word length suggested that AR's reading was often based on a serial process. High frequency words were read with a rate of 133 ms/letter. However, this reduced to 70 ms/letter when the data were reanalysed with outliers >3000 ms removed. The rate for semantic decisions, also cleaned of outliers, was 187 ms/letter. Slow serial processing was also observed for responses to non-words in the lexical decision and vocalisation experiments. These rates appear generally to be somewhat above those found among the competent readers.

Table 7.4 gives the results from the visual matching tasks. Identity matching was achieved with reaction time levels and error rates which lay within the normal range. Array matching RTs, on the other hand, were well above 2000 ms and were widely dispersed. This suggests that AR's visual processor functioned normally at the level of identity matching but that there was some disturbance at the level of parsing and analytic comparison. There were no consistent effects of orthographic legality. The positions of difference functions were not indicative of any consistent use of a slow left-to-right processing strategy.

		Semantic decisions		
Typical positives	Atypical positives	Related negatives	Unrelated negatives	All
1863	1691	2489	2079	2013
1528	729	1309	1164	1268
0	20^3	26.67^3	7.14	13.56
				136

TABLE 7.4   *Reaction times (ms) and error rates for visual matching tasks*

Experiment		Identity matching			Array matching	
		Overall	Rate (ms/letter)		Overall	Position of difference (ms/position)
1	X̄	1004	32[1]	X̄	2261	127
	sd	460		sd	1019	
	Error %	1.67		Error %	4	
2	X̄	1110	7	X̄	2838	316[1]
	sd	465		sd	1691	
	Error %	1.85		Error %	9.17	
3	X̄	1009	9	X̄	2766	106
	sd	373		sd	1072	
	Error %	0		Error %	6.88	

[1] Linear trend significant at $p < 0.05$ or better by F-test

TABLE 7.5   *Reaction times (ms) and error rates for reading normal and distorted words or non-words by AR*

		Vocalisation tasks		Decision tasks	
		Words	Non-words	Semantic	Lexical
Normal	X̄	1094	1830	1573	1390
	sd	465	999	628	432
	Error %	0	23.33	2.08	8.33
	Rate	129[1]	−13	74	150[1]
Zigzag	X̄	1397[2]	2701	1786	1861[2]
	sd	616	2387	579	706
	Error %	3.33	10	4.26	16.67
	Rate	276[1]	662[1]	156[1]	210[1]
Vertical	X̄	1520[2]	2516	1999[2]	1810[2]
	sd	515	1768	651	615
	Error %	0	10	6.52	6.67
	Rate	125[1]	548[1]	219[1]	235[1]

[1] Significant linear trend
[2] Format effect on reaction time
[3] Format effect on accuracy

The format distortion effects have been summarised in Table 7.5, and appear somewhat variable. If word reading is considered, AR's performance is within the normal range for all cases except responses to low frequency zigzag words. AR appears to have been quite strongly affected by the zigzag distortion which produced processing rates equal to or slower than the rates for vertical words in a number of instances. Very slow processing rates were associated with non-word reading in the vocalisation tasks and the lexical decision tasks.

3   Conclusions

AR's Level I (competence) description indicates that he is an individual of above average intelligence who experienced difficulties in acquiring reading and spelling skills during primary schooling. The effect on spelling was somewhat more severe than the effect on reading.

The Level II (cognitive) description has been summarised in Table 7.6. The overall impression is one of a diffuse impairment affecting the visual processor and the morphemic routes. AR's non-word reading was relatively efficient and showed some sophistication in the use of higher order correspondences. The effects on the morphemic routes principally took the form of occasional delayed responses, although there was also evidence of serial reading. This could imply an impairment of the wholistic mode of the visual processor which is relatively more damaging for the morphemic routes than for route 'g'. The difficulty with zigzag distortions might fit in with this account. At the same time, AR's slowness in array matching is indicative of an impairment of the analytic mode of the processor, and the lack of clear position of difference effects suggests that he did not operate a systematic serial processing strategy in comparison.

TABLE 7.6.   *Summary of cognitive description of reading functions of subject AR*

Function	Status	Comment
'm' → phonology	Mild effect	Large frequency effect. Semantic and grapheme-phoneme support. Fast serial processing
'g' → phonology	Mild effect	Use of major correspondences. Errors on complex vowels. Serial processing
'm' → scmantics	Mild effect on decision time	Effects of frequency, typicality and relatedness on accuracy. Serial processing
Visual processor	Impaired	Slow array matching. Slow format resolution for non-words

Case II.2   Laurence A (born November 1968)

1   Psycho-educational background

Laurence had an 'at risk' birth (an emergency Caesarian section following a prolonged labour). His progress during the first 6 months was followed by the neonatal clinic but no problems were noted. Early developmental milestones were said to have been normal. He walked at 14 months and had a substantial vocabulary by 22 months. He was brought up in a literate environment and was frequently read to and encouraged to take an interest in books and general matters. The first indications of possible learning difficulties appeared when he was in the Primary 2 class. His teacher questioned whether he was seeing the blackboard properly and arranged for a sight test. Shortly afterwards she commented that he might have problems in motor co-ordination which made it difficult for him to write. Remedial teaching was arranged. His school reports noted difficulty in reading and writing, and commented on a lack of concentration and distractability. In Primary 3, Laurence's mother became concerned that he was falling seriously behind in reading and number work and becoming tense and unhappy at school. His reading and attempts at writing were characterised by reversals and inversions. Number sequences were confused and were sometimes written from right to left with mirror image digits. Private tuition with an educational psychologist was arranged and found to be helpful. The school did not respond positively to the suggestion, put by Laurence's mother, that he might be 'dyslexic'. She requested an investigation by the Child Guidance Service and at the same time arranged for an assessment from the local dyslexia association. The reports tended to agree that Laurence was of above average intelligence, that he was behind in his reading, and that he was noticeably distractable. There were references to problems of visual memory and 'faulty scanning' and also poor spelling and handwriting. When Laurence reached the age for transfer to secondary school his parents decided that he should attend a school in Edinburgh which offered specialised facilities for the teaching of dyslexic children. With the assistance of a scribe he passed five 'O' Grade examinations and is now preparing to sit five subjects at the Higher Grade. He is interested in music and reads four or five books for pleasure each year.

LA's general intelligence was assessed by means of the WISC-R at the ages of 7 years, 11 years and 15 years. The results, summarised in Table 7.7, consistently show above average performance on the verbal and performance scales. Scaled sub-test scores for the 1984 administration have been included in the table. The psychologist noted a depression on the arithmetic and digit span verbal tests which she considered to be part of 'a characteristic dyslexic pattern in which there is some impairment of the short-term sequential auditory memory'. The marked drop on the coding sub-test was considered to indicate a 'very specific difficulty with written output'. The observation that this test also involves perception of the orientation of abstract shapes and that the block design score was somewhat lower than the other performance scales was considered to point to the possibility of a visual functional difficulty.

LA's reading competence was formally tested at intervals throughout his school career. Table 7.8 summarises the results of these various tests. The Neale test typically indicated that comprehension was at or ahead of chronological age although the rate and accuracy scores were depressed. Overall, a progression towards a competent level of performance in reading

TABLE 7.7   *Results of administration of the WISC to subject LA (a) in 1976 when subject's CA was 7-2 years, (b) in 1976 when subject's CA was 7-9 years, (c) in 1979 when subject's CA was 11 years, and (d) in 1984 when subject's CA was 15-10 years*

	Verbal tests		Performance tests	
	Information	13	Picture completion	11
	Comprehension	16	Picture arrangement	16
	Arithmetic	7	Block design	14
a	Similarities	9	Object assembly	14
	Vocabulary	13	Coding	11
	Digit span	8		
	Verbal IQ 111		Performance IQ 124	
	Arithmetic	8	Block design	15
	Similarities	13	Object assembly	13
b	Vocabulary	13		
	Digit span	8		
	Verbal IQ 124		Performance IQ 135	
	Information	11	Picture completion	11
	Similarities	16	Picture arrangement	12
	Arithmetic	13	Block design	15
c	Vocabulary	16	Object assembly	15
	Comprehension	13	Mazes	10
	Digit span	12		
	Verbal IQ 122		Performance IQ 118	
	Information	12	Picture completion	14
	Similarities	13	Picture arrangement	14
	Arithmetic	10	Block design	12
d	Vocabulary	16	Object assembly	17
	Comprehension	15	Coding	9
	Digit span	10		
	Verbal IQ 119		Performance IQ 123	

is evident. In some of the earlier reports, LA's reading was described as 'intelligent guesswork' and as involving 'many visual errors because of over-fast and inaccurate word processing'. In the 1984 assessment there were errors involving letter sequence, omission and insertion of sounds, and sound-symbol mismatches. Comprehension under timed conditions was poorer than under untimed conditions and this was considered to be a consequence of LA's technical difficulties in reading. Non-word reading gave a score of 18/22 which was thought to suggest a slight problem in phonological processing.

As mentioned above, spelling and writing were considered to be a major difficulty for LA from the very beginnings of his primary schooling. An example of free writing produced at the age of 8 years appears to be typical

TABLE 7.8　*Results of formal tests of reading competence for subject LA*

Age	Test	Result	
7-2　years	Daniels and Diack Standard Reading Test 1	5-9　years	
7-3　years	Daniels and Diack Standard Reading Test 1	5-7　years	
7-3　years	Daniels and Diack Test 2	6-9　years	
7-9　years	Neale Analysis of Reading Ability	6-0　years:	rate
		7-0　years:	accuracy
		7-3　years:	comprehension
		7-8　years:	rate
8-6　years	Neale Analysis of Reading Ability	7-11　years:	accuracy
		9-1　years:	comprehension
		7-7　years:	rate
9-7　years	Neale Analysis of Reading Ability	8-2　years:	accuracy
		12-1　years:	comprehension
10-8　years	Daniels and Diack Test 12 (reading comprehension)	11-6　years	
10-8　years	Burt Re-arranged Word Reading Test	10-3　years	
		9-6　years:	rate
11-0　years	Neale Analysis of Reading Ability	10-1　years:	accuracy
		12-4　years:	comprehension
12-11 years	Schonell Graded Word Reading Test	12-4　years	
15-10 years	Schonell Graded Word Reading Test A	13-6　years	
15-10 years	Daniels and Diack Test 12 (reading comprehension)	13-7　years	
15-10 years	Schonell Silent Reading Test (R4) B	11-9　years	

'dyslexic writing', showing oddities of format and letter formation and a mixture of partially phonetic and seemingly 'bizarre' spellings. Table 7.9 details the results of spelling tests applied at intervals between the ages of 7 years and 15 years. A marked retardation is evident in every instance. A report by an educational psychologist in 1979 noted that his writing was executed over-hastily and that his spelling errors were phonetically accurate but inconsistent. In 1980 his teacher reported success in overcoming negative attitudes to writing and in establishing some fundamental spelling rules. In 1984, his writing was described as poorly formed, with inappropriate grasp and angle of the pencil, incorrect use of capitals, absence of punctuation and poor spelling. Occasional b-d reversals were found in his schoolwork. The content of his writing was described as imaginative and the expression as satisfactory.

In 1976, LA, then aged 7-2 years, completed the Illinois Test of Psycholinguistic Abilities and obtained a composite age of 7-3 years, with good scores on the auditory sub-tests. An articulatory confusion between /f/ and /θ/ was noted. Application of the Lindamood Auditory Conceptualisa-

TABLE 7.9   *Results of spelling tests administered to LA*

Age	Test	Result
7-3 years	Daniels and Diack Spelling Test	6-0 years
9-7 years	Daniels and Diack Spelling Test	7-3 years
10-6 years	Daniels and Diack Spelling Test	8-1 years
10-8 years	Vernon Spelling Test	7-5 years
11-0 years	Daniels and Diack Spelling Test	7-9 years
12-11 years	Schonell Spelling Test	8-8 years
15-10 years	Schonell Graded Word Spelling Test A	10-4 years

tion test in 1984 gave a score of 88/100. The psychologist considered that this revealed some weakness in the ability to reflect on and compare the identity, number and sequence of sounds in words, although she did not think that the problem was sufficiently marked to account for LA's difficulties.

Various efforts were made to assess LA's visual functions. A report in 1976 mentioned poor performance on tasks involving the copying of arrays of shapes. An administration of the Aston Index the following year indicated a depressed score on the test of visual sequential memory for symbolic material. In 1984, orthoptics testing using the Dunlop procedure suggested the absence of a stable reference eye and treatment involving the occlusion of the left eye was recommended and undertaken. The score on the Graham Kendall Memory for Designs test was described as perfect and this was taken as an indication that LA's visual difficulties were print-specific.

The various items from the Bangor Dyslexia test were administered in 1984. LA obtained a score of 5, which was regarded as significant. He encountered difficulties in left-right discrimination, repetition of poly-syllables, and the recall of the multiplication tables and the months sequence. Problems in learning to tie shoelaces and to read the clock were also reported. The persistence of b-d confusions has already been mentioned.

2   Experimental data

LA was tested by C. Porpodas when he was aged 8-7 years. His results at that time were suggestive of a combined morphemic and phonological dyslexia. Non-words were slowly read (the mean VRT was over 3000 ms) and there were errors on more than 30 per cent of trials. Word reading was also slow, with VRTs between 2000-3000 ms and numerous errors on items of irregular spelling. For high frequency words, irregularity increased error rate from 6 per cent to 42 per cent.

The results from the present series of experiments, applied when LA was aged 13 years, appear in Table 7.10. The reaction time distributions have been plotted in Figure 7.2. All three distributions contain a preponderance of times below 2000 ms together with a tail of slower responses (Type B distributions). There was no major differentiation between high frequency words and low frequency words or between words and non-words.

TABLE 7.10   *Vocal reaction times (ms) and error rates for reading high frequency words, low frequency words and non-words by LA*

	High frequency words			Low frequency words			Non-words		
	Overall	Intercept	Slope	Overall	Intercept	Slope	Overall	Intercept	Slope
$\bar{X}$	1399	942	96	1797	516	273[1]	1910	593	278
sd	1200			1698			2700		
Error %	4.79			11.11			22.46		

[1] Linear trend significant at p<0.02 or better by F-test
Frequency effect: t(269) = 2.252, p<0.025. $\chi^2(1)$ = 4.131, p<0.05
Lexicality effect (HF v NW):t(340) = 2.198, p<0.025. $\chi^2(1)$ = 23.764, p<0.001
       (LF v NW):t(293) = 0.396. $\chi^2(1)$ = 7.012, p<0.01

LA's results for non-word reading are suggestive of a mild phonological effect. The error rate was somewhat high (22 per cent) and the reaction time distribution included occasional slow responses. The homophony variation had no effect. However, about 20 per cent of responses showed evidence of the use of higher order correspondences and this 'lexicalisation score' approached 44 per cent for the subset of items drawn from consistently irregular environments. These results suggest that LA's translation channel operated on sophisticated correspondences but without reference to the speech production lexicon.

The word reading data show an elevation of error rates and reaction time levels together with a number of slow responses. There was a significant effect of frequency on error rate and a reaction time effect of almost 400 ms. These data are indicative of a mild impairment of the morphemic route to phonology.

LA's word reading was affected by the semantic/syntactic factors. The reaction time to read function words was greater by 500 ms than the mean for high frequency content words and there was a delay of about 100 ms in the reading of low frequency abstract words (p<0.05 in both cases). This suggests an involvement of semantic processing in word retrieval. There was also evidence of phonological effects. Irregularity increased error rate for low frequency words from 3.57 to 25 per cent (p<0.05). A number of errors appeared to be phonetic regularisations (e.g. muscle → 'muskel', key → 'kay', prove read to rhyme with 'grove'). These data suggest that the grapheme-phoneme channel was also involved in the reading of less familiar words.

The results from the lexical decision tasks have been summarised in

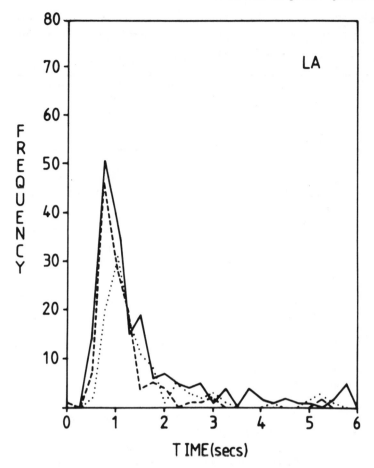

FIGURE 7.2 *Reaction time distributions for responses to high frequency words (– – –), low frequency words (. . .) and non-words (——) by LA*

Table 7.11. The reaction time levels were within the normal range, although discrimination between low frequency words and legal non-words was poor. Frequency effects on positive decisions were inconsistent but there were reliable effects of legality on the accuracy and latency of negative decisions. Results from the semantic decision experiment appear in Table 7.12. Performance was relatively accurate (11.86 per cent of errors) but the reaction time was elevated (2546 ms) and the distribution was widely dispersed with a long tail of slow responses. There were large reaction time effects of typicality and relatedness. Some slowing in the process of accessing and operating on semantic information seems to be indicated.

TABLE 7.11　*Reaction time (ms) and error data from four lexical decision experiments by LA*

Experiment		HF words	LF words	Legal non-words	Illegal non-words	All
1	$\bar{X}$	1054	1354[2]	1603	1126	1177
	sd	417	675	1008	570	610
	Error %	0	13.64[3]	60[3]	0	12.4
	Rate (ms/letter)		−37	237	64	32
2	$\bar{X}$	1041	1172	1174[2]	1015	1091
	sd	404	399	429	305	388
	Error %	15.56	24.44	35.16[3]	4.44	20
	Rate (ms/letter)	−	−	−	−	58[1]
3	$\bar{X}$	815	918	1088[2]	726	878
	sd	333	301	318	211	321
	Error %	12.5	12.5	17.02[2]	2.08	10.99
4	$\bar{X}$	8.23	894	1074	811	888
	sd	285	247	394	154	294
	Error %	8.33	30.56	30.56	5.56	18.75

[1] Significant linear trend
[2] Significant effect on reaction time
[3] Significant effect on error rate

TABLE 7.12　*Reaction time (ms) and error data for semantic decisions by LA*

	Typical positives	Atypical positives	Related negatives	Unrelated negatives	All
$\bar{X}$	1930	2842[2]	3198[2]	2245	2546
sd	1035	1293	1613	1144	1384
Error %	13.33	17.86	10	6.67	11.86
Rate (ms/letter)					106

[1] Significant linear trend
[2] Significant effect on reaction time
[3] Significant effect on accuracy

The results of the matching experiments, summarised in Table 7.13, were not suggestive of a major visual processor impairment. Identity judgments were made with a fast reaction time and parallel processing of the letter arrays. There was no evident delay in the array matching experiments. The orthographic legality effect was not significant in the standard experiment, although there was an effect in one of the subsidiary experiments.

TABLE 7.13   *Reaction times (ms) and error rates for visual matching tasks by LA*

Experiment		Identity matching				Array matching	
		Overall	Rate (ms/letter)			Overall	Position of difference (ms/position)
1	$\overline{\text{X}}$	606	1		$\overline{\text{X}}$	1011	100[1]
	sd	126			sd	320	
	Error %	8.33			Error %	23	
2	$\overline{\text{X}}$	683	8		$\overline{\text{X}}$	1616	249[1]
	sd	207			sd	883	
	Error %	16.05			Error %	14.17	
3	$\overline{\text{X}}$	644	5		$\overline{\text{X}}$	1604	23
	sd	179			sd	695	
	Error %	1.67			Error %	6.29	

[1] Linear trend significant at $p < 0.05$ or better by F-test

There were some indications of serial left-to-right processing, but with rates which were within the normal range. The one feature of the matching performance which stands out is the occurrence of atypically high error rates in the second identity matching experiment and in the first array matching experiment.

The effects of word length in the vocalisation and decision experiments have been included in the tables. The data do not give strong indications of serial processing. The linear trend tests were not significant for the lexical decision and semantic decision tasks. The word reading data, analysed with outliers >3000 ms removed, gave a rate of 70 ms/letter for high frequency words. The effect on non-word reading was not significant.

Table 7.14 suggests that LA's reading was also relatively unaffected by the format distortion manipulation. The distortions did not modify the processing rates in the lexical and semantic decision tasks. In the vocalisation experiments there was a large effect of vertical distortion on non-word reading and an effect of zigzag distortion of low frequency word reading. High frequency words were relatively unaffected.

3   Conclusions

LA's case has been the subject of frequent formal assessments. These support a Level I description which identifies him as an individual of above average ability and originality who has suffered severe difficulties in developing spelling, writing and reading skills. The reports suggest an accompanying short-term memory deficit and visual problems relating to direction and orientation which are possibly attributable to the failure to establish a stable reference eye.

TABLE 7.14   *Reaction times (ms) and error rates for reading normal and distorted words or non-words by LA*

		Vocalisation tasks		Decision tasks	
		Words	Non-words	Semantic	Lexical
Normal	X̄	939	1317	1387	1020
	sd	256	616	668	386
	Error %	3.33	16.67	10.64	16.67
	Rate	36	95	98	37
Zigzag	X̄	1595^2	2185^2	1366	1220^2
	sd	600	1754	510	441
	Error %	3.33	26.67	25.53	16.67
	Rate	215^1	−15	81	76^1
Vertical	X̄	1254^2	2115^2	1418	1026
	sd	441	1217	501	271
	Error %	6.67	33.33	14.58	26.67
	Rate	60	497^1	37	71^1

[1] Significant linear trend
[2] Format effect on reaction time
[3] Format effect on accuracy

The Level II (cognitive) description is indicative of a combined mild morphemic and phonological dyslexia. The conclusions have been summarised in Table 7.15. A balanced effect of this kind could plausibly derive from a visual disorder which had the effect of degrading position and identity information about letters. However, such an effect would be expected to influence performance on the matching and distortion resolution tasks, and it is consequently surprising that the experimental analysis does not give clearer evidence of visual processor impairments.

TABLE 7.15   *Summary of cognitive description of reading functions of subject LA*

Function	Status	Comment
'm' → phonology	Mild effect	Large frequency effect. Function word effect. Semantic and grapheme-phoneme support
'g' → phonology	Mild effect	Use of major correspondences
'm' → semantics	Mild effect	Slow semantic decisions. Large typicality and relatedness effects
Visual processor	Efficient	High error rates in identity matching and array matching. Fast serial processing in array matching

LA shares with AR a description in which the morphemic and grapheme-phoneme translation routes are mildly affected to an approximately equal degree and both semantic processes and grapheme-phoneme translation are used as back-up procedures during word retrieval. A further common factor is the relative sophistication of the translation channel. LA differs from AR in that he does not give clear evidence of serial reading or of effects on the analytic functions of the visual processor.

Case II.3   Scott M (born July 1968)

1   Psycho-educational background

Scott's birth was reported to have been normal. No delays in passing early developmental milestones were noted although his speech was slightly defective and required therapy. He was not a clumsy child and learned to tie his shoelaces before going to school. His hearing and vision were tested at about 6 years and were found to be normal. No behaviour problems were reported. His father was said to have had difficulties with spelling. Scott was referred for assessment to the Tayside Dyslexia Association in 1980. He received remedial tuition in school and also some private tuition through the Association.

An intellectual assessment was carried out in 1980 using the Wechsler scales. This indicated an average intelligence level with a fairly marked verbal-performance discrepancy (Verbal IQ = 94, Performance IQ = 117). His reading and spelling were both impaired. Reading age, assessed by the Neale tests, was 7-5 years for rate, 9 years for accuracy and 11-4 years for comprehension. His spelling age was 8-3 years on the Daniels and Diack test. A reassessment, carried out in 1981 using the Schonell tests, suggested a substantial improvement (reading age = 11-2 years, spelling age = 9-6 years).

2   Experimental data

A summary of SM's results for reading high frequency words, low frequency words and non-words appears in Table 7.16. The reaction time distributions are displayed in Figure 7.3. The results are suggestive of a combined morphemic and phonological impairment. A phonological dyslexia is indicated by the high error rate on non-word reading (27 per cent) and by the dispersed appearance of the distribution. The morphemic dyslexia is marked by the rise in error rate on low frequency words to almost 24 per cent, by elevation of the reaction time level, and by the presence, in the distributions for both high and low frequency words, of an extended tail of slow responses. The frequency effect was about 400 ms. There were significant differences between high and low frequency words but not between low frequency words and non-words.

The analysis of the effects of the psycholinguistic factors revealed no effect of form class, although abstract meaning was associated with a small

TABLE 7.16   *Vocal reaction times (ms) and error rates for reading high frequency words, low frequency words and non-words by SM*

| | High frequency words | | | Low frequency words | | | Non-words | | |
	Overall	Intercept	Slope	Overall	Intercept	Slope	Overall	Intercept	Slope
X̄	1490	348	243[1]	1906	699	268[1]	2023	445	331[1]
sd	775			977			819		
Error %	5.99			23.81			27.12		

[1] Linear trend significant at p<0.05 or better by F-test

Frequency effect: $t(251) = 3.727$, p<0.001. $\chi^2(1) = 19.849$, p<0.001

Lexicality effect (HF v NW):$t(327) = 6.026$, p<0.001. $\chi^2(1) = 29.129$, p<0.001

(LF v NW):$t(266) = 1.041$, $\chi^2(1) < 1$

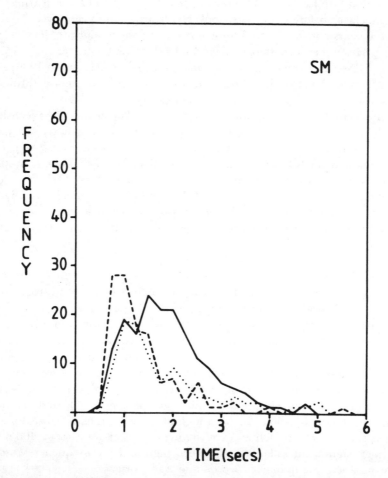

FIGURE 7.3   *Reaction time distributions for responses to high frequency words (– – –), low frequency words (. . .) and non-words (———) by SM*

TABLE 7.17 *Reaction times (ms) and error rates for reading regular and irregular words of high and low frequency by SM*

| | High frequency words | | Low frequency words | |
	Regular	Irregular	Regular	Irregular
$\bar{\text{X}}$	1402	1553	1919	2813[1]
sd	519	781	711	1254
Error %	3.57	14.29	7.14	53.57[2]

[1] Significant effect on reaction time
[2] Significant effect on accuracy

rise in error rate. The effects of spelling-to-sound irregularity were much more substantial and have been documented in Table 7.17. For low frequency words the error rate rose to over 50 per cent and there was a rise in reaction time of nearly 900 ms. These results suggest a reliance on grapheme-phoneme translation during word reading. This conclusion is supported by a consideration of SM's errors which included several phonetic regularisations. These have been listed in Table 7.18.

TABLE 7.18 *Examples of phonetic regularisation errors produced by SM*

Target	Response	Target	Response	Target	Response
heir	/hɛə/	whereby	/wəbɪ/	aisle	/ɑsəl/
corps	/kɔəps/	average	/eɪvəreɪdz/	isle	/ɪsəl/
bomb	/bu:m/	honour	/hɒnɒə/		
		grief	/graɪf/		
		ache	/ətʃ/		
		mow	/mɔəwə/		
		cousin	/ku:zɪn/		

The results from the non-word reading experiments suggested that SM's grapheme-phoneme channel operated without reference to the speech production lexicon. Homophony affected neither reaction time nor accuracy. On the other hand, some responses to non-words gave evidence of the use of higher level correspondences (e.g. rasten → /reɪsən/, squant → /skwɒnt/, sprild → /spraɪld/). This lexicalisation score was about 17 per cent. The initial /w/ rule was applied on 4 out of 6 occasions. Thus, SM shares with AR and LA a tendency to make use of some correspondences above the grapheme-phoneme level.

SM's error responses were words and non-words with about equal frequencies. The latencies showed an advantage for word responses. The errors were generally structurally close to their targets (average similarity = 67 per cent), and showed a typical tendency for mistakes to occur on the complex structures, especially the vowels.

TABLE 7.19   *Reaction time (ms) and error data for lexical and semantic decisions by SM*

	HF words	LF words	Lexical decisions Legal non-words	Illegal non-words	All
$\bar{\text{X}}$	1380	1855^2	2071	1850	1729
sd	530	960	585	615	703
Error %	5.26	18.18	20	0^3	8.33
Rate (ms/letter)	270^1		349^1	53	201^1

[1] Significant linear trend
[2] Significant effect on reaction time
[3] Significant effect on error rate

The efficiency of route 'm' to semantics was assessed by considering the results from the decision experiments. The data have been summarised in Table 7.19. Semantic decisions were accurately made, but the reaction time level was elevated and the distribution very dispersed. This constitutes evidence for an effect on the process of accessing and using semantic information. There were no clear effects of relatedness or typicality.

The lexical decision results have been included in the table. These also show some exaggeration of the reaction time level and a wide dispersion of the distribution. There were effects of legality on accuracy and of frequency on reaction time in the standard experiment but the pattern of these effects varied from one experiment to another.

The analysis of SM's visual processor functions gave very clear evidence of serial letter-by-letter reading. The length effects for the vocalisation and decision tasks have been included in Tables 7.16 and 7.19. In each case reaction time was related to word length by a linear function having a slope of 200 ms/letter or more. The rates for responses to non-words were in excess of 300 ms/letter. These functions were all strongly significant on a linear trend test and appear extremely regular. Reanalyses following removal of outlying reaction times did not alter this conclusion.

Results from the visual matching tasks have been summarised in Table 7.20. Matching of pairs of letter arrays was achieved accurately but with an elevated reaction time and further indications of serial processing. There was a significant left-to-right trend in the standard experiment with a slope of 287 ms/position and a rate of over 400 ms/letter in the experiment using horizontal and vertical displays. These data suggest the involvement of a serial self-terminating process with a slow functional rate. There was a 200 ms effect of orthographic legality on positive decisions. Identity matching appears to have been performed accurately and with a reaction time well within the normal range, although two of the experiments showed effects of variations in the number of letters presented for matching.

| | Semantic decisions | | | |
Typical positives	Atypical positives	Related negatives	Unrelated negatives	All
1433	1789[2]	2375	2367	1997
574	904	746	886	884
6.67	10.71	10	3.33	7.63
				223[1]

TABLE 7.20   *Reaction times (ms) and error rates for visual matching tasks by SM*

| Experiment | | Identity matching | | | Array matching | |
		Overall	Rate (ms/letter)		Overall	Position of difference (ms/position)
1	$\bar{\text{X}}$	812	18[1]	$\bar{\text{X}}$	1499	287[1]
	sd	228		sd	453	
	Error %	2.5		Error %	8	
2	$\bar{\text{X}}$	960	21[1]	$\bar{\text{X}}$	2157	425[1]
	sd	259		sd	590	
	Error %	2.47		Error %	6.67	
3	$\bar{\text{X}}$	876	0	$\bar{\text{X}}$	2290	197[1]
	sd	207		sd	692	
	Error %	1.67		Error %	1.88	

[1] Linear trend significant at $p < 0.05$ or better by F-test

These results suggest that SM's visual processor typically operated in a slow serial mode. If the effect of format distortions is to force a switch to this mode, then it is possible that no large effects of distortion will be found in an individual who is already committed to serial processing. The summary of the distortion data contained in Table 7.21 gives some support to this suggestion. In the semantic decision experiment the processing rates were in excess of 300 ms/letter for the normal format as well as for the distorted items. A similar outcome occurred for the reading of high frequency words. In the other cases the serial functions observed for normal presentation were apparently exaggerated by the distortions.

TABLE 7.21   *Reaction times (ms) and error rates for reading normal and distorted words or non-words by SM*

| | | Vocalisation tasks | | Decision tasks | |
		Words	Non-words	Words	Non-words
Normal	X̄	1672	1897	1745	1750
	sd	841	781	996	912
Error %		6.67	26.67	4.17	13.33
	Rate	342[1]	231[1]	352[1]	149
Zigzag	X̄	2253	2532[2]	2181[2]	2547[2]
	sd	1967	815	1357	1518
Error %		6.67	20	6.52	16.67
	Rate	557[1]	308[1]	392[1]	529[1]
Vertical	X̄	2396[1]	2318	2254[2]	2465[2]
	sd	1464	1301	1086	954
Error %		6.67	44.83	0	25
	Rate	483[1]	544[1]	389	274[1]

[1] Significant linear trend
[2] Format effect on reaction time
[3] Format effect on accuracy

3   Conclusions

SM's Level I description identifies him as a boy with above average non-verbal intelligence who has suffered difficulties in developing a basic competence in reading and spelling. A possible involvement of early speech difficulties is also indicated.

The Level I (cognitive) description suggests the presence of a fairly evenly balanced set of impairments affecting the morphemic routes and

TABLE 7.22   *Summary of cognitive description of reading functions of subject SM*

Function	Status	Comment
'm' → phonology	Impaired	High error rate on low frequency words. Large frequency effect. Large regularity effect on low frequency words. Phonetic regularisations. Slow serial processing
'g' → phonology	Impaired	Some use of major correspondences. Difficulty with complex vowels. Slow serial processing
'm' → semantics	Effect on decision time	Serial processing
Visual processor	Impaired wholistic function	Orthographic model. Slow serial process in matching. Slow format resolution

ɔneme translation combined with an impairment of the
de of the visual processor. These conclusions have been
n Table 7.22. The two novel features in SM's case are (1) the
f the effect of spelling-to-sound irregularity on low frequency
, and (2) the restriction to slow serial reading across a range of
. These results suggest an impairment of the capacity of the
sor to parse letter arrays wholistically or by a fast serial
visual processing defect is accompanied by a reliance on
ɩoneme translation when reading unfamiliar words, producing
ʏslexic' pattern of the kind described by Coltheart *et al.* (1983).

Graham S (born June 1968)

educational background

s the first born of twin brothers. Pregnancy and delivery were
ve been normal. No family history of learning disability was
He was an unsettled baby who cried a lot during his first
He did not crawl, but walking and early language development
dered to have been normal. Mastery of shoelace tying and
clock were thought to have been a bit late. His health in
was satisfactory apart from a period in hospital at the age of
ɩe to psoriasis. The primary school he attended was generally
ɩc to his problems. He received tuition through the Tayside
ssociation for about three years up to the age of 13 years which
ɩed to have been helpful. He left secondary school at the age of
ʏout taking any 'O' Grades. After a period on a youth training
ɩok up an apprenticeship as a cycle mechanic. His hobbies are
cycling and football. He reads a local newspaper but does not
s at all.
ɩment of his general intelligence when he was aged 8 years
abbreviated WISC) suggested above average verbal ability
vith below average performance ability (Verbal IQ = 121,
e IQ = 83). A reassessment in 1984, using the WAIS, gave the
s shown in Table 7.23. These results do not confirm the earlier
of a verbal-performance discrepancy.
s reading was assessed by the Neale test at the age of 8-4 years.
ɔn all three measures were then just under a year behind his
ɩl age. A further test, at the age of 12-9 years, using the Daniels
graded test of reading experience, gave a reading age of 12-
ɩ administration of the Schonell test in 1981 gave a less
result (reading age = 10-4 years). When he was tested again in
ɔre had risen to 12-5 years. His performance on an untimed test
ɔmprehension (Daniels and Diack test 12) was good (age = 13-

TABLE 7.23   *Results of the administration to GS (a) of WISC tests in 1976 when subject's CA was 8 years, and (b) of WAIS tests in 1985 when subject's CA was 16-7 years*

	Verbal scores		Performance scores	
a	Verbal IQ	121	Performance IQ	83
b	Information	9	Digit symbol	13
	Comprehension	9	Picture completion	14
	Arithmetic	10	Block design	10
	Similarities	9	Picture arrangement	9
	Digit span	9	Object assembly	9
	Vocabulary	11		
	Verbal IQ	102	Performance IQ	108

7 years) but he did poorly on the Schonell timed test (age = 9-8 years). This was considered to be an effect of the slowness of his reading. His score on a test of reading nonsense syllables was 19/22.

Tests of spelling revealed a consistent impairment. When tested in 1981 his score on the Daniels and Diack test was 9-2 years, while his score on the Schonell test was 8-5 years. By 1984 this had risen to 10-4 years. The psychologist commented that his errors were mostly phonetically plausible attempts. In free composition he produced looped cursive handwriting with heavy pen pressure. The volume of output and expression were regarded as satisfactory, although the spelling and punctuation were weak.

GS's score on the items from the Bangor test was 3/10, which was not considered to be significant. He made errors in the reverse digit sequence, repetition of polysyllables, left-right discrimination and the reverse months sequence. His performance on the Graham Kendall Memory for Designs test suggested no impairment of visual shape memory. On the other hand, his score on the Lindamood Auditory Conceptualisation test was only 64/100. The psychologist reported that this score was indicative of a serious weakness in the ability to manipulate the sounds in words. She commented that this poor score was surprising in the light of GS's relatively good performance in nonsense syllable reading. On the Lindamood test he was very poor at representing the sounds of nonsense syllables by manipulation of a sequence of coloured blocks, although his performance with single sounds suggested that phonemic discrimination was not a problem.

2   Experimental data

GS's results for reading high frequency words, low frequency words and non-words are shown in Table 7.24. It can be seen that low frequency words were less accurately and more slowly read than either high frequency words or non-words. The pattern is in general consistent with the presence

TABLE 7.24   *Vocal reaction times (ms) and error rates for reading high frequency words, low frequency words and non-words by GS*

| | High frequency words | | | Low frequency words | | | Non-words | | |
	Overall	Intercept	Slope	Overall	Intercept	Slope	Overall	Intercept	Slope
$\bar{x}$	1695	455	264[1]	2562	571	427[1]	2292	405	389[1]
sd	782			1817			1063		
Error %	9.52			24.6			13.14		

[1] Linear trend significant at p<0.05 or better by F-test

Frequency effect: t(245) = 5.145, p<0.01. $\chi^2(1)$ = 12.19, p<0.002

Lexicality effect (HF v NW):t(355) = 5.831, p<0.001. $\chi^2(1)$ = 1.245

(LF v NW):t(298) = 1.608. $\chi^2(1)$ = 7.611, p<0.01

of a morphemic dyslexia accompanied by a relatively less severe phonological dyslexia.

A morphemic dyslexia is suggested by the high error rates in word reading (10 per cent for high frequency words, 25 per cent for low frequency words), by the relatively high reaction time levels, and by the large effects of word frequency (frequency effect = 867 ms). The vocal reaction time distributions, displayed in Figure 7.4, show that there were a number of slow responses to high frequency words and that the distribution for low frequency words was widely dispersed with a long tail of very slow responses.

The main evidence for the presence of a phonological dyslexia is given by the reaction time level in non-word reading (nearly 2300 ms) and by the wide dispersion of the non-word distribution. The error level, at 13 per cent, was within the range of the competent reader sample. This rate was not significantly greater than the rate for high frequency words and was significantly *lower* than the rate for low frequency words. The observation that GS read non-words more accurately than low frequency words is consistent with the suggestion that his primary impairment is morphemic rather than phonological. Non-words were also read faster than low frequency words, although in this case the difference was not quite significant.

A configuration in which a severe morphemic impairment is accompanied by a relatively milder phonological effect is expected to result in a reliance on route 'g' when reading unfamiliar words, giving rise to regularity effects and regularisation errors. Table 7.25 shows that GS's accuracy of reading lower frequency words was very strongly affected by spelling-to-sound regularity. Irregularity increased error rate from 11 per cent to 68 per cent although there was no effect on reaction time. The syntactic factor (form class) had no effect and the effects of abstract meaning were limited to a small impact on accuracy of reading high frequency words. Table 7.26 lists the errors made by GS which appeared to

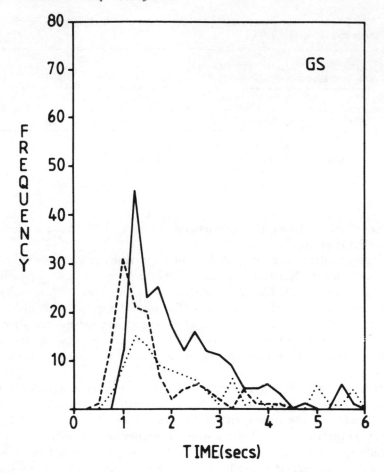

FIGURE 7.4   *Reaction time distributions for responses to high frequency words (– – –), low frequency words (. . .) and non-words (———) by GS*

be phonetic regularisations. The occurrence of these errors together with the large effect of irregularity on low frequency word reading supports the conclusion that GS relied on the grapheme-phoneme translation channel when reading unfamiliar words.

The analysis of non-word reading suggested that GS attempted to lexicalise output from the grapheme-phoneme channel. Homophony reduced error rate from 17 per cent to 5 per cent and speeded vocal reaction time by about 400 ms (p<0.05). The results from the experiment varying lexical environment indicated that about 17 per cent of responses showed evidence of the use of major correspondences (e.g. molf → /mɑlf/, wamp → /wɒmp/, thost → /θoɔst/). For items from the consistently irregular set the lexicalisation score was about 28 per cent. This suggests

TABLE 7.25 *Reaction times (ms) and error rates for reading regular and irregular words of high and low frequency by GS*

	High frequency words		Low frequency words	
	Regular	Irregular	Regular	Irregular
$\overline{X}$	1539	1744	2542	2043
sd	694	921	2087	1418
Error %	0	7.14	10.71	67.86[2]

[1] Significant effect on reaction time.
[2] Significant effect on accuracy.

TABLE 7.26 *Examples of phonetic regularisation errors produced by GS*

Target	Response	Target	Response
through	/θrɔʊ/	society	/sɒkɪtɪ:/
corps	/kɔəps/	canoe	/kænɔʊ/
comb	/kʌm/	plough	/plɔʊ/
laugh	/lɔə/	muscle	/mʌskəl/
heir	/hɪə/	isle	/ɪsəl/

that GS operated a relatively sophisticated translation channel and that its output was referred to the speech production lexicon.

The frequencies and latencies of word and non-word error responses are shown in Table 7.27. GS's responses were both words and non-words although there was a tendency for target and response lexicality to covary (p<0.05). Non-word responses to words were made particularly slowly. The errors were generally structurally similar to their targets (average similarity = 69 per cent) and usually involved minor misapplications of correspondence rules and positioning errors. Complex vowels were most frequently mistranslated.

TABLE 7.27 *Frequencies and latencies (ms) of error responses to word and non-word targets by GS*

	Word		Non-word	
	Word	Non-word	Word	Non-word
$\overline{X}$	3187	6336	2507	2629
Sd	2813	5220	1503	1334
N	30	17	11	20

Table 7.28 provides a summary of the results from the semantic decision task. Performance was relatively accurate (11 per cent of errors) although with a large effect of typicality. The reaction time level was elevated at over

TABLE 7.28   *Reaction times (ms) and error rates for semantic decisions by GS*

	Typical positives	Atypical positives	Related negatives	Unrelated negatives	All
$\overline{\text{X}}$	1701	1944	2327	2261	2065
sd	737	717	488	653	703
Error %	3.33	31.03[3]	10	0	10.92
Rate (ms/letter)					139[1]

[1] Significant linear trend
[2] Significant effect on reaction time
[3] Significant effect on accuracy

2000 ms and the distribution showed wide dispersion. Some impairment of the process of accessing and operating on semantic information is suggested.

Table 7.29 contains the results from four lexical decision experiments. The data are rather variable. In the first experiment, the reaction time level was slightly elevated (over 1600 ms) and the distribution contained a tail of slow responses, mainly contributed by the legal non-words. The error rate on low frequency words was very high at over 40 per cent. The other experiments all showed strong effects of legality and high rates of error on either low frequency words or legal non-words. Taken together, these results are indicative of an impairment of the morphemic route affecting both decision time and accuracy of discrimination of unfamiliar vocabulary.

In the case of subject SM, the morphemic impairment appeared to be associated with a tendency to read by a slow serial letter-by-letter procedure having a rate of 200 or more ms/letter. GS did not show this effect in the decision tasks. There was no significant linear component in responses to words in the lexical decision task and the rate of 139 ms/letter observed for semantic decisions was slow but within the normal range for the task. The length effects in the vocalisation tasks have been summarised in Table 7.23. These rates were generally slower than 200 ms/letter, and the linear trends were strongly significant. For high frequency words, a rate of 264 ms/letter remained virtually unchanged when outlying reaction times were removed from the distribution. Removal of outliers reduced the rate for low frequency words from 427 ms/letter to 157 ms/letter. Non-word reading was achieved by a very slow serial process, having a rate of 389 ms/letter. These results indicate that the operation of route 'm' to phonology was based on a slow serial process but that this was not also true of route 'm' to semantics.

The results from the matching experiments, summarised in Table 7.30, do not appear indicative of a general impairment of the visual processor. Reaction times and error levels for identity judgments were well within the

TABLE 7.29   *Reaction time (ms) and error data for lexical decisions by GS*

	HF words	LF words	Legal non-words	Illegal non-words	All
X̄	1513	1812	2457	1305^2	1616
sd	701	564	1137	736	875
Error %	7.89	40.91^3	20^3	0	13.33
Rate (ms/letter)		90	519^1	225^1	197^1
X̄	1580	2253^2	2238^2	1858	1946
sd	615	1288	957	752	932
Error %	17.78	46.67^3	24.44^3	4.44	23.33
Rate (ms/letter)	–	–	–	–	226^1
X̄	1202	1686^2	1586^2	1234	1405
sd	571	839	682	410	668
Error %	6.25	16.67	31.25^3	2.08	4.06
X̄	1731	2037	3504^2	16.21	2071
sd	1026	1104	1952	536	1322
Error %	11.11	11.11	47.22^3	5.56	18.75

[1] Significant linear trend
[2] Significant effect on reaction time
[3] Significant effect on error rate

TABLE 7.30   *Reaction times (ms) and error rates for visual matching tasks by GS*

Experiment		Identity matching Overall	Rate (ms/letter)		Array matching Overall	Position of difference (ms/position)
1	X̄	825	15^1	X̄	1735	229^1
	sd	248		sd	489	
	Error %	0.83		Error %	10	
2	X̄	973	24^1	X̄	2045	221^1
	sd	375		sd	586	
	Error %	2.47		Error %	5	
3	X̄	877	3	X̄	1840	93^1
	sd	330		sd	577	
	Error %	0.83		Error %	2.5	

[1] Linear trend significant at $p<0.05$ or better by F-test

normal range although there was evidence of length effects in the standard experiment and for vertical displays in the experiment varying format of presentation. Array matching was within the normal range for the main experiment. There was an orthographic legality effect of over 300 ms. The

TABLE 7.31   *Reaction times (ms) and error rates for reading normal and distorted words or non-words by GS*

		Vocalisation tasks		Decision tasks	
		Words	Non-words	Semantic	Lexical
Normal	X̄	2393	2874	1912	1734
	sd	1381	1362	678	846
Error %		3.33	20	10.42	20
	Rate	454[1]	245	19	118
Zigzag	X̄	2263	3363	2088	2019
	sd	1442	2005	943	902
Error %		10	20	20.83	18.33
	Rate	531[1]	838[1]	149	286[1]
Vertical	X̄	2275	3963[2]	2155	2106[2]
	sd	1329	2563	754	1013
Error %		6.67	16.67	12.5	31.67
	Rate	323[1]	1084[1]	217[1]	301[1]

[1] Significant linear trend
[2] Format effect on reaction time
[3] Format effect on accuracy

position of difference function suggested the involvement of serial processing with a rate of about 230 ms/position.

The format distortion effects have been summarised in Table 7.31. The effects were within the normal range for semantic decisions and were somewhat variable for the other tasks. There were large effects on the vocalisation of words but these occurred for normally formatted displays as well as for distorted displays.

3   Conclusions

GS's Level I description identifies him as an individual of average ability whose academic achievements have been limited as a consequence of dyslexic difficulties in reading and spelling. The test results are discrepant but give evidence of problems in spatial manipulation at one stage and of conceptualisation of phonemic elements at another.

The Level II (cognitive) description has been summarised in Table 7.32. The striking feature is an effect on route 'm' to phonology which appears relatively more severe than the accompanying effects on route 'g' or route 'm' to semantics. The visual processor operates in a slow serial mode when attempting to access phonology and this process is supported by grapheme-phoneme translation via a relatively accurate and sophisticated channel. The grapheme-phoneme channel appears, in its turn, to rely on support from the lexical system when organising a response.

TABLE 7.32 *Summary of cognitive description of reading functions of subject GS*

Function	Status	Comment
'm' → phonology	Impaired	Large frequency effect. Large regularity effect on low frequency words. Phonetic regularisations. Slow serial processing
'g' → phonology	Impaired	Lexicalisation. Some use of major correspondences. Difficulty with complex vowels. Slow serial processing
'm' → semantics	Impaired	Typicality effect. Frequency effect
Visual processor	Impaired wholistic function	Orthographic model. Serial processing. Slow format resolution, especially in vocalisation tasks

Case III.5   Lesley H (born August 1970)

1   Psycho-educational background

Lesley H is an example of a girl who would not be accepted as 'dyslexic' if exclusionary criteria were applied, since she has low general intelligence, comes from a disadvantaged background, and has a disrupted educational history.

Her mother reported that her birth had been normal. It was thought that early speech development may have been delayed. The home background was disturbed with the father periodically in prison. An older sibling died as a result of a glue sniffing tragedy. Lesley's early schooling was in a city in the north of England and was disrupted by frequent moves. Her teachers attributed her difficulties with reading and spelling to this disruption and to laziness and unwillingness to work. Her mother suspected learning difficulties when Lesley was about 8 years old. When the family returned to Scotland in 1979 she approached the Tayside Dyslexia Association and arranged for an assessment. Thereafter small group remedial teaching was provided daily. Her school reports praised her diligence and application but noted her difficulties with English. Her mother said that she spent considerable time on her homework each evening and that she was 'a bright girl, but she feels it not being able to keep up with the rest of the class'. Lesley herself commented that her peers at school 'mak´ a fool o´ us' on account of her low marks. She enjoys swimming and karate and playing outdoor games like hide-and-seek but does not read for pleasure. She is left-handed. Her mother stated that she had had spelling difficulties herself.

An intellectual assessment carried out on behalf of the Association in 1979 suggested poor verbal intelligence (Verbal IQ = 67, Performance IQ = 96). A new assessment in 1984 confirmed this conclusion, giving the scaled WISC scores shown in Table 7.33. The psychologist commented on the rather even pattern of sub-test scores and the marked depression of language functions. The low verbal scores contrasted with LH's chatty and communicative manner although the content of what she said was described as not always logical or to the point.

TABLE 7.33 *Results of administration of the WISC to subject LH in 1984*

Verbal tests		Performance tests	
Information	2	Picture completion	9
Similarities	5	Picture arrangement	9
Arithmetic	5	Block design	9
Vocabulary	5	Object assembly	9
Comprehension	6	Coding	7
Digit span	6		
Verbal IQ	67	Performance IQ	90

TABLE 7.34 *Results of administration of reading and spelling tests to LH in 1984 when subject's CA was 14-2 years*

Reading ages		Spelling ages	
Schonell (test A)	9-6 yrs	Schonell (test A)	9-6 yrs
Daniels and Diack (test 12)	10-7 yrs		
Schonell (R4 test)	8-10 yrs		

The results of assessments of LH's reading and spelling undertaken in 1984 are shown in Table 7.34. A general impairment is indicated in both cases. It was noted that she sub-vocalised audibly when carrying out the silent comprehension test. She scored 17/22 on a test of nonsense word reading, suggesting only a mild degree of impairment of phonological assembly. Her spelling errors were often phonetically plausible attempts. As a left-hander she held the page at 90 degrees while writing. Her free composition contained examples of grammatical errors, lack of punctuation, inappropriate capitalisation, poor sentence structure and repetitive expression. The psychologist noted that her spelling and reading ages were approximately equivalent.

Auditory discrimination was tested in 1979 using the Wepman test. No impairment was noted. In 1984 she scored 83/100 on the Lindamood Auditory Conceptualisation test. The psychologist commented that this score was predictive of difficulties in a middle primary school child although she did not consider that the errors made by LH were suggestive of severe difficulties in auditory conceptualisation. The Graham Kendall Memory for Designs test, administered in 1984, gave no evidence of an impairment of visual memory for shapes. However, orthoptics testing carried out in the same year suggested the possibility that LH had not established a stable reference eye. The Bangor Dyslexia test gave a score of 9, with difficulties evident in left-right discrimination, repetition of polysyllables, recall of the tables, reversed months sequence and digit span. There was one error in reading the clock face. LH reported that she still occasionally reversed 'b' and 'd'.

2 Experimental data

The reaction time and accuracy data for reading high frequency words, low frequency words and non-words are displayed in Table 7.35. Figure 7.5 shows the reaction time distributions for correct responses. The data appear indicative of a combined morphemic and phonological dyslexia.

TABLE 7.35 *Reaction times (ms) and error rates for reading high frequency words, low frequency words and non-words by LH*

| | High frequency words | | | Low frequency words | | | Non-words | | |
	Overall	Intercept	Slope	Overall	Intercept	Slope	Overall	Intercept	Slope
$\bar{X}$	2205	−320	539[1]	2761	815	420[1]	2566	745	368[1]
sd	2206			2093			1411		
Error %	21.43			44.88			25.42		

[1] Linear trend significant at $p < 0.05$ or better by F-test
Frequency effect: $t(200) = 1.726$, $p < 0.05$. $\chi^2(1) = 18.429$, $p < 0.001$
Lexicality effect (HF v NW): $t(306) = 1.74$, $p < 0.05$. $\chi^2(1) = 0.865$
               (LF v NW): $t(244) = 0.841$. $\chi^2(1) = 14.312$, $p < 0.001$

The phonological dyslexia is marked by a fairly high error rate in non-word reading (25 per cent) and by an elevated reaction time and dispersed distribution. Non-word reading was not affected by homophony but a high proportion of responses (about 30 per cent) involved the use of higher order correspondences (e.g. gind → /gaɪnd/). These data suggest that LH read non-words via a relatively sophisticated translation channel which operated without reference to the speech production lexicon.

LH's morphemic dyslexia is marked by a high error rate and dispersed reaction time distribution for reading both high and low frequency words. The high frequency word distribution includes a tail of very slow responses and the low frequency distribution lacks a preponderance of fast responses. The word frequency effect was 556 ms. The reaction time difference between low frequency words and non-words was not significant and the error rate for non-words was significantly lower. On these grounds, it can be argued that LH's phonological impairment is relatively less severe than her morphemic impairment.

A configuration of this kind is expected to result in a reliance on route 'g' during reading, producing regularity effects and regularisation errors.

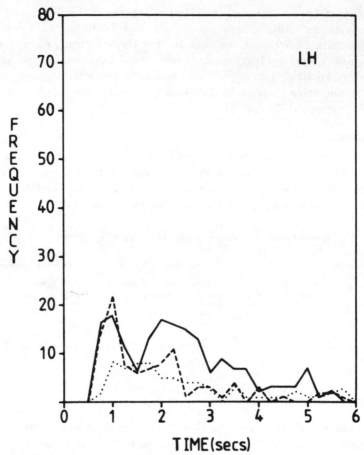

FIGURE 7.5 *Reaction time distributions for responses to high frequency words (– – –), low frequency words (. . .) and non-words (———) by LH*

Table 7.36 contains the data from the experiment in which spelling-to-sound regularity was varied. Irregularity had no effect on reaction time but large effects on accuracy for both high and low frequency words. The error rate for low frequency irregular items was over 60 per cent. More than 20 of LH's error responses appeared to involve phonetic regularisation. Examples have been listed in Table 7.37 and include standard responses such as sew → 'sue' and blood → 'blude'.

The data from the experiment varying syntactic/semantic factors suggested that there were no effects due to form class but that abstract meaning had a large influence on the latency of responses to high frequency words (1835 ms versus 3545 ms, p<0.01 by t-test). This effect suggests some involvement of semantic processes in retrieving responses to familiar words.

TABLE 7.36 *Reaction times (ms) and error rates for reading regular and irregular words of high and low frequency by LH*

	High frequency words		Low frequency words	
	Regular	Irregular	Regular	Irregular
$\bar{X}$	2025	2053	2206	2212
sd	1145	1481	1108	788
Error %	10.71	35.71[2]	28.57	67.86[2]

[1] Significant effect on reaction time
[2] Significant effect on accuracy

TABLE 7.37 *Examples of phonetic regularisation errors produced by LH*

Target	Response	Target	Response	Target	Response
heir	/hɪə/	whereby	/wɛəbɪ/	aisle	/eɪsəl/
ski	/skaɪ/	benefit	/bnɪːfɪt/	hymn	/aɪmen/
sew	/suː/	machine	/mæettʃɪn/	ache	/eɪʃ/
tongue	/tɒŋ/	anger	/əendzə/	isle	/ɪsəl/
comb	/kʌm/	agony	/eɪgɒnɪ/		
bough	/boʊ/	canoe	/kæenoʊ/		
corps	/kɔəps/	blood	/bluːd/		
muscle	/muːsɪkəl/	scene	/skɛn/		
ewe	/əweɪ/	debt	/dɛpt/		

LH's results from the lexical and semantic decision tasks suggested that route 'm' to semantics was also impaired. The reaction time distribution for semantic decisions has been plotted in Figure 7.6 and can be seen to be widely dispersed and to lack a preponderance of fast times. The mean RT

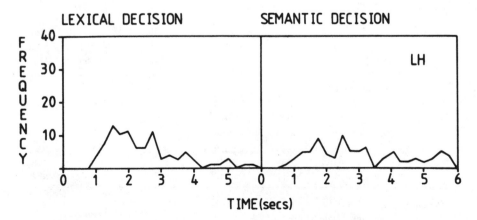

FIGURE 7.6   *Reaction time distributions for lexical and semantic decisions by LH*

was over 3000 ms and there were numerous errors (27 per cent overall) especially in classification of atypical positives (43 per cent of errors) or related negatives (31 per cent of errors). These results, shown in Table 7.38, are suggestive of severe difficulties in retrieval and use of semantic information.

TABLE 7.38   *Reaction time (ms) and error data for semantic decisions by LH*

	Typical positives	Atypical positives	Related negatives	Unrelated negatives	All
$\bar{X}$	2321	2567	4501	4007	3396
sd	1180	1355	1577	2263	1928
Error %	23.33	42.86	31.03	13.33	27.35
Rate (ms/letter)					407[1]

[1] Significant linear trend
[2] Significant effect on reaction time
[3] Significant effect on accuracy

TABLE 7.39   *Reaction time (ms) and error data for lexical decisions by LH*

Experiment		HF words	LF words	Legal non-words	Illegal non-words	All
1	$\bar{X}$	2012	2502	2960	3129	2630
	sd	746	1227	1010	1553	1302
	Error %	13.16	36.36[3]	35[3]	10	20
	Rate (ms/letter)		218	549[1]	186	229
2	$\bar{X}$	2319	2597	2652	2840	2598
	sd	940	1204	1298	1404	1236
	Error %	15.56	40[3]	37.78[3]	15.56	27.22
	Rate (ms/letter)	–	–	–	–	285[1]
3	$\bar{X}$	2009	2486[2]	2711	2968	2505
	sd	801	940	1444	1547	1242
	Error %	2.13	14.89[3]	54.17[3]	14.58	21.58
4	$\bar{X}$	2392	2570	2834	2594	2565
	sd	909	1238	1051	1360	1165
	Error %	11.11	33.33[3]	52.78[3]	16.67	28.47

[1] Significant linear trend
[2] Significant effect on reaction time
[3] Significant effect on error rate

Figure 7.6 also shows the distribution for lexical decisions. This too was widely dispersed and included numerous slow responses. The mean scores from four experiments, shown in Table 7.39, indicate that the RTs were delayed for words and non-words alike and that there were generally no clear effects of either word frequency or legality. Error levels tended to be high on the low frequency items and the legal non-words, indicating poor discrimination of less familiar vocabulary.

These results show that LH was poor at recognising lower frequency items but she did possess information about orthographic structure which was helpful to her in making negative decisions. Indeed, she commented of the vowel-less non-words that they couldn't be words because they did not include 'proper letters'.

The results from the visual matching experiments have been summarised in Table 7.40. Identity matching was performed accurately and with a reaction time which was at the upper end of the normal range. Mean reaction time in array matching, on the other hand, showed large delays which are suggestive of an impairment of the analytic function of the visual processor. There was evidence of slow serial processing in the experiment using horizontal and vertical formats but not in the other two experiments. The legality effect was almost 700 ms in the standard experiment.

TABLE 7.40   *Reaction times (ms) and error rates for visual matching tasks by LH*

Experiment		Identity matching			Array matching	
		Overall	Rate (ms/letter)		Overall	Position of difference (ms/position)
1	$\bar{X}$	1131	21[1]	$\bar{X}$	3163	−93
	sd	365		sd	1182	
	Error %	0		Error %	2	
2	$\bar{X}$	1223	9	$\bar{X}$	2956	448[1]
	sd	499		sd	1547	
	Error %	2.47		Error %	3.33	
3	$\bar{X}$	844	−3	$\bar{X}$	2507	−23
	sd	171		sd	734	
	Error %	0		Error %	2.5	

[1] Linear trend significant at $p < .05$ or better by F-test

Like SM and GS, LH's reading appears to have involved a slow serial procedure. Her processing rates were 400 ms/letter for semantic decisions and 368 ms/letter for non-word reading. A rate of over 500 ms/letter for reading high frequency words was reduced to 200 ms/letter when outlying responses >400 ms were removed but the linear trend remained strongly significant. These results suggest an impairment of the wholistic function of the visual processor which caused all three major routes to operate on the basis of slow letter-by-letter processing.

Table 7.4 gives the results from the format distortion experiments. The general impression is that a serial processing procedure was adopted for normal and distorted displays alike. Thus, in reading words aloud the processing rate was over 600 ms/letter for the normal format and 500-500 ms/letter for the distortions. In non-word reading and in semantic decisions the distortions appeared to further delay an already slow and serial process.

TABLE 7.41   *Reaction times (ms) and error rates for reading normal and distorted words or non-words by LH*

		Vocalisation tasks		Decision tasks	
		Words	Non-words	Semantic	Lexical
Normal	$\overline{X}$	2414	2297	2913	2325
	sd	1386	693	1315	1003
Error %		3.33	20	14.89	26.67
	Rate	639^1	174^1	283^1	221^1
Zigzag	$\overline{X}$	2467	3217^2	2809	2687
	sd	1154	1485	1442	1458
Error %		30^3	26.67	16.67	23.33
	Rate	403^1	611^1	445^1	285^1
Vertical	$\overline{X}$	3122^2	3548	3306	2793^2
	sd	1391	1736	1563	1153
Error %		10	26.67	21.28	31.67
	Rate	503^1	684^1	516^1	355^1

[1] Significant linear trend
[2] Format effect on reaction time
[3] Format effect on accuracy

Overall, the implication is that LH's visual processor was impaired with respect to the availability of a wholistic processing facility and the rate of operation of an analytic procedure.

3   Conclusions

LH's Level I description identifies her as a girl of below average intelligence, especially in the verbal domain, who has suffered some social and educational disadvantages and whose performance in reading and spelling has been consistently poor for her age.

The Level II description suggests the presence of impairments in all major system, including: (1) effects on the wholistic and analytic modes of the visual processor, (2) large effects on the morphemic routes to semantics and phonology, and (3) a relatively less severe effect on route 'g' to phonology. These conclusions have been summarised in Table 7.42. It seems very probable that LH's poor verbal intelligence, reflecting an impoverishment of the conceptual structures available within the semantic processor and a restriction on the range of vocabulary represented within the phonological processor, will have contributed to the impairment of the morphemic routes. Some features of her performance, such as the effect of abstract meaning on high frequency word reading and the high error rate on atypical items in the categorisation task, seem consistent with this view.

TABLE 7.42   *Summary of cognitive description of reading functions of subject LH*

Function	Status	Comment
'm' → phonology	Impaired	Large frequency effect. Large regularity effect. Effect of abstract meaning. Phonetic regularisations. Slow serial processing
'g' → phonology	Impaired	Use of major correspondences. Slow serial processing
'm' → semantics	Impaired	Slow responses. Errors on atypical items and related negatives. Poor discrimination in lexical decisions. Slow serial processing
Visual processor	Impaired	Orthographic model. Slow matching. Slow format resolution

7.3   Conclusions

The subjects included in Series III gave greater evidence of morphemic impairments than those placed in Series I and II. In addition, I excluded from the series those subjects who combined a morphemic impairment with a major phonological effect. The results should, therefore, be illustrative of the data which might be expected from a 'surface dyslexic' configuration, that is one in which damage to the 'm' routes occurs in the context of a relative sparing of the 'g' route.

The Series III subjects differed in the severity of the morphemic effect they demonstrated. In subjects AR and LA the effect was quite mild with error rates on lower frequency words falling below 12 per cent. The other three subjects all showed more substantial effects on error rates and reaction times.

AR and LA exhibited a set of mild generalised impairments and are, in this respect, similar to the Series II subjects, DP and DT. LA differs from AR chiefly in the lack of evidence of visual processor effects. Features such as slow serial processing, slow array matching and slow resolution of distortions appeared in the data of AR but not LA. The results from the tests of central functions suggested fairly evenly balanced effects on the three routes, with some evidence of sophistication in the translation route (indexed by the use of V+C correspondences in non-word reading) and a tendency to support word retrieval by semantic processes as well as grapheme-phoneme translation (shown by semantic and phonological effects on word reading).

The remaining three subjects, SM, GS and LH, showed more severe morphemic effects. Their reading of words was marked by slow responses and high error rates, especially for items of low frequency. The effects were more substantial for subject LH who was both younger and less intellectually able than SM and GS. For this reason it seems sensible to consider SM and GS together and to treat LH separately.

SM and GS exhibited some common features. The operation of route 'm' to phonology was characterised by (1) a large effect of word frequency on reaction time and error rate, (2) a large effect of spelling-to-sound irregularity on the accuracy of reading lower frequency words, (3) the occurrence of appreciable numbers of phonetically regularised errors, and (4) the reading of words by a slow serial process having a rate of about 200 ms/letter. A point of difference between them is that regularity affected both accuracy and reaction time in the case of GS but accuracy only in the case of SM. The two subjects also showed small effects of abstract meaning on reading accuracy. These results are consistent with the proposal that the establishment of words in a morpheme recognition system was limited for words of lower frequency (and possibly items of more abstract meaning) and that the translation channel played a critical role in support of word retrieval.

Both SM and GS showed evidence of an impairment of route 'g'. There was an effect on accuracy and translation time for SM but on translation time alone for GS. These results, taken together with those of the other subjects who show some morphemic effects (e.g. FM, AR and LA), suggest that a morphemic effect will usually be accompanied by some effects on grapheme-phoneme translation. This conclusion contrasts with the proposal for impairments of route 'g', since the data of JK and JS in the competent reader sample, and of AD and SS in Series I, indicated that an effect on route 'g' did not necessarily compromise the morphemic routes. It is of course possible that future research will discover cases in which a morphemic impairment is combined with the efficient operation of route 'g'. However, this configuration did not present itself in the present sample.

Both subjects read non-words by a serial procedure. They also gave evidence of the availability of information about orthographic structure within the visual processor and of the use of some correspondences above the level of simple grapheme-phoneme associations. This suggests that their non-word reading involved a consideration of segments larger than single letters and that their translation channels were, in this sense, sophisticated or lexicalised. The two subjects differed in their readiness to refer output from the translator to the speech production lexicon. The analysis of homophony effects suggested that this was done by GS but not by SM. Both subjects were liable to error in vowel translation and both produced a mixture of word and non-word error responses. The observation that neologisms did not predominate implies that the errors were not exclusively products of a defective translation process. Thus, SM and GS's reading can be seen as involving an occasional reliance on the translation process but not an exclusive dependence on that process.

Both subjects also showed a measure of impairment of route 'm' to semantics. This concurrence has appeared in the data of all of the other subjects showing an effect on route 'm' to phonology and suggests that morphemic effects are likely to extend to both routes. Nonetheless, the effect was relatively mild and SM and GS were differentiated in terms of the degree of dependence of the semantic route on serial processing. SM appeared to read serially in the semantic tasks as well as in the vocalisation tasks, whereas for GS serial reading occurred only when vocalisation was required.

This latter distinction has implications for the analysis of visual processor functions in morphemic dyslexia. If the dyslexia derived from a general impairment of the wholistic function of the visual processor, then serial processing should be evident in all reading tasks. SM's data are consistent with an analysis of this kind. The observation that GS relied on letter-by-letter processing in the vocalisation tasks but not in the decision tasks implies that the serial processing may be an adaptation to the demands of the higher level systems rather than a property of the visual processor itself.

For LH, the analysis of the morphemic dyslexia is complicated by the need to evaluate the contribution of her low IQ. Poor verbal intelligence could affect reading development in a number of ways: (1) it might limit the capacity to isolate and associate phonemic segments and their graphemic equivalents; (2) a restriction on the range of vocabulary represented in the phonological processor might limit the range of words which could be recognised by route 'm' to phonology; (3) a restriction on the complexity of the conceptual structures available to the semantic processor might limit the range of words which could be recognised within route 'm' to semantics. It is, in addition, possible that a low level of verbal intelligence could be associated with a diffuse inefficiency, resulting in slow or inaccurate information processing over a wide range of cognitive tasks.

The possibility of a generalised processing inefficiency can be examined by considering the data from the identity matching experiments. LH's reactions in this task were accurate and no slower than those of much more intelligent children.

The low IQ appears not to have been responsible for a particular impairment of route 'g'. LH's non-word reading was slow and liable to error but no more so than several older subjects of much higher intelligence. Further, the legality effects observed in the lexical decision and array matching experiments suggested that she had abstracted information about orthographic structure while her use of higher order correspondences in non-word reading indicated that she had established a relatively sophisticated translation channel.

Nonetheless, LH's range of reading vocabulary was severely curtailed when considered relative to the other subjects who have been discussed. Regularity affected high frequency words as well as low frequency words indicating that even relatively common words required grapheme-phoneme support for response retrieval. The large effects of abstract meaning suggested the involvement of a semantic system in which abstract items were poorly represented. The effects of typicality and relatedness in the semantic decision experiment also suggested limitations on the resources or precision of the semantic processor.

8 Series IV and V: phonological dyslexia

8.1 Introduction

In Chapter 7 I presented the results for five dyslexic cases in whom a morphemic impairment was combined with a relatively mild phonological disturbance. In this chapter I propose to consider eight more cases who all showed quite large phonological effects. Their results should provide an opportunity to analyse the consequences of serious inefficiency in grapheme-phoneme translation processes. On these grounds I have entitled this chapter 'phonological dyslexia', although I would emphasise that all of the cases to be considered had some accompanying morphemic impairments. The contrast, therefore, is between cases of morphemic dyslexia having a small phonological effect (the Series III subjects) and those having a large effect.

For convenience of presentation I have divided this group into two subsets. Series IV included three subjects (JM, SE and MP) in whom the phonological effect on either accuracy or reaction time fell within or close to the range encompassed by the competent reader group. The Series V subjects (SB, LT, MT, JB and PS) all showed very large effects on both accuracy and reaction time.

According to the standard theory, the effect of a severe impairment of route 'g' should be to discourage the use of grapheme-phoneme translation while favouring the use of semantic processing. Hence, severe phonological disturbances might be expected to be accompanied by a diminution in regularity effects and the occurrence of some semantic effects.

8.2 Series IV case studies: mild phonological effect

Series IV included three male subjects. JM was an adolescent of average or above average general ability. SE and MP were young adults. SE was of average ability whereas MP was well below average, especially in the

169

performance area.

The order in which the cases are presented has been determined by their reaction time levels for reading high frequency words.

Case IV.1   James M (born August 1967)

1   Psycho-educational background

James M was born without complication, the sixth of six children. No family history of learning disability was reported. He was hospitalised at 4 months on account of gasto-enteritis when he suffered dehydration and convulsions. Developmental milestones were reported as normal apart from absence of crawling and some delay of speech onset. Tying of shoelaces and mastery of the clock did not present any particular difficulties. At school, a learning problem was evident in the Primary 1 class. He spent the whole year with the same reading book and became very reluctant to attend school. When matters had not improved by the Primary 3 class remedial tuition was arranged. The referral to the Tayside Dyslexia Association in 1976 was on the advice of his class teacher. The extra tuition was discontinued after JM's transfer to secondary school. He passed five subjects at the 'O' Grade (Chemistry, Physics, Arithmetic, Modern Studies and Technical Drawing) but failed English and Mathematics. A spelling concession was allowed. After leaving school he obtained a position as an architect's technician and began attending a day release course at a Technical College. He reported that he still had difficulty in making notes and in reading back what he had written afterwards. He is a keen football supporter and enjoys computer games. He reads a newspaper but never reads books for pleasure.

JM's general abilities were assessed in 1976. Scores on an abbreviated WISC were suggestive of an average level of intelligence. A further assessment, using the WAIS, was undertaken in 1984 and gave the scaled scores shown in Table 8.1. These place JM's intelligence above the average. The psychologist commented that the low score on the arithmetic sub-test was a characteristic dyslexic feature although it was not, in this instance, accompanied by a poor score on the digit span tests. The low score on the digit-symbol test was seen as being consistent with slow writing and handling of symbols. A relative reduction in the scores on picture completion and object assembly by contrast with the very good performance on block design and picture arrangement was considered to imply a possible difficulty in figure-ground perception.

JM's reading abililties were tested in 1976, 1981 and 1984. The results, summarised in Table 8.2, show that at the age of 9 years he was about one year behind his age in reading but that the gap had widened slightly by 1981. His scores for 1984 indicate that he had obtained reading ages above

TABLE 8.1 *Results of administration of the WAIS to subject JM in 1984*

Verbal tests		Performance tests	
Information	11	Digit symbol	9
Comprehension	14	Picture completion	12
Arithmetic	8	Block design	15
Similarities	15	Picture arrangement	16
Digit span	12	Object assembly	12
Vocabulary	11		
Verbal IQ	116	Performance IQ	120

TABLE 8.2 *Results of administration of tests to subject JM (a) in 1976 when subject's CA was 9-4 years, (b) in 1979 when subject's CA was 11-9 years, (c) in 1981 when subject's CA was 14-1 years, and (d) in 1984 when subject's CA was 17-4 years*

	Reading ages		Spelling ages	
a	Neale Analysis		Daniels and Diack	
	rate	8-2 years		7-7 years
	accuracy	8-0 years		
	comprehension	9-1 years		
b	British Abilities Scale		Daniels and Diack	
		10-7 years		10-2 years
c	Schonell Graded Word		Schonell Graded Word	
		11-4 years		10-8 years
d	Schonell (test A)		Schonell (test A)	
		13-1 years		10-8 years
	Daniels and Diack (test 12)			
		13-7 years		
	Schonell (R4 test)			
		11-9 years		

13 years in word recognition and untimed comprehension. The lower score on the timed comprehension test was attributed to his slowness in reading. On a test of reading nonsense syllables he scored only 14/22 which was taken to indicate a serious weakness in phonological assembly.

The results of formal assessments of JM's spelling have been included in Table 8.2. These indicate that he consistently fell behind his age in spelling and that there was no real progress between 1981 and 1984. The educational psychologist commented on the phonetic nature of some of his errors and also noted that he had a confusion in speech between /b/ and /r/ which appeared in some of his spelling errors. He himself commented that he tended to make more errors in continuous writing. A sample of free writing obtained in 1984 contained numerous spelling mistakes with poor punctuation, expression and grammar. The psychologist noted that his grasp of the pencil was incorrect and that some letters, especially 'f', were poorly formed.

JM's record contains various references to speech-related difficulties, including delayed language development and a tendency to be mixed up over sounds, although he appears not to have been referred to a speech therapist at any stage. In 1984 his score on the Lindamood test was 73/100 which was considered to be indicative of a serious weakness in the ability to reflect on and compare the identity, number and sequence of sounds in words.

No evidence of an impairment of visual memory was given by the Graham Kendall test. His score on the items from the Bangor test was within the range of Miles's dyslexic group, chiefly on account of difficulty in left-right discrimination, repetition of polysyllables and recall of multiplication tables.

2   Experimental data

JM participated in the studies carried out by C. Porpodas in 1976-77 when he was aged about 10 years. His results at that time were suggestive of a combined phonological and morphemic dyslexia. Non-word reading was somewhat inaccurate (27 per cent of errors) and very slow (VRT = 4600 ms). Words were also read slowly, with a latency of about 3000 ms, and there was a strong effect of word frequency. Spelling-to-sound irregularity had a large effect on accuracy of reading lower frequency words, raising error rate from 10 per cent to 46 per cent. Lexical decisions were slow, with a latency over 3500 ms, and there were numerous failures to recognise words (39 per cent of errors on positive trials).

The analysis of JM's reading carried out in 1981-82 suggests a persistence of the phonological dyslexia and a progression towards resolution of the morphemic dyslexia. The data for reading non-words and words of high and low frequency have been summarised in Table 8.3. Distributions of reaction times are presented in Figure 8.1. A 'phonological dyslexia' is indicated by the high error rate in non-word reading (over 30 per cent) and by the widely dispersed distribution of reaction times. Non-word reading was differentiated from low frequency word reading in terms of both accuracy and reaction time. The lexicality effect was 685 ms.

The persistence of the 'morphemic dyslexia' is suggested by the elevated error rates for reading both high and low frequency words and the large word frequency effects. The distributions contain a predominance of times in the faster range, but there is in each case a tail of slower responses and these are more numerous for low frequency than for high frequency words.

The analysis of the effects of the psycholinguistic variables established that there were no form class effects but that abstract meaning caused an

TABLE 8.3   *Vocal reaction times (ms) and error rates for reading high frequency words, low frequency words and non-words by JM*

| | High frequency words | | | Low frequency words | | | Non-words | | |
	Overall	Intercept	Slope	Overall	Intercept	Slope	Overall	Intercept	Slope
X̄	1209	434	164[1]	1603	429	257[1]	2288	−3	474[1]
sd	743			1161			1275		
Error %	10.2			20.78			30.51		

[1] Linear trend significant at $p<0.05$ or better by F-test

Frequency effect: $t(296) = 3.556$, $p<0.001$. $\chi^2(1) = 7.624$, $p<0.01$

Lexicality effect (HF v NW):$t(338) = 9.58$, $p<0.001$. $\chi^2(1) = 26.337$, $p<0.001$
 (LF v NW):$t(284) = 4.649$, $p<0.001$. $\chi^2(1) = 4.511$, $p<0.05$

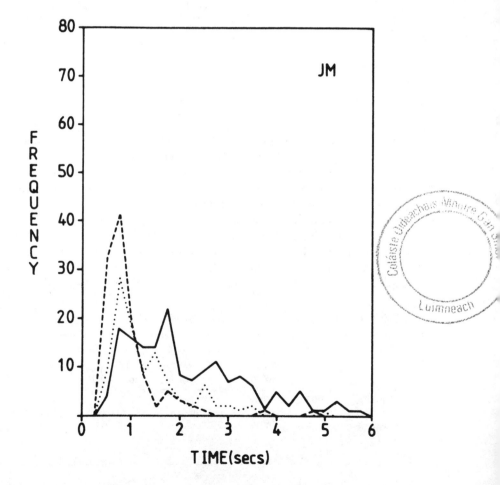

FIGURE 8.1   Reaction time distributions for responses to high frequency words (– – –), low frequency words (. . .) and non-words (——) by JM

overall reaction time delay of about 500 ms (p<0.05). The effects of spelling-to-sound irregularity have been summarised in Table 8.4. There were no reaction time effects, but irregularity increased error rate on low frequency items from 7 per cent to 35 per cent. The abstraction effect suggests the involvement of some semantic back-up processing. The effect of regularity indicates that, despite the phonological dyslexia, grapheme-phoneme translation was used to support word retrieval.

TABLE 8.4   *Reaction times (ms) and error rates for reading regular and irregular words of high and low frequency by JM*

	High frequency words		Low frequency words	
	Regular	Irregular	Regular	Irregular
$\overline{X}$	899	914	1147	1285
sd	353	286	483	650
Error %	7.14	7.14	7.14	35.71[2]

[1] Significant effect on reaction time
[2] Significant effect on accuracy

The reaction time in non-word reading was reduced from 2600 ms to about 2000 ms by homophony (p<0.05). This implies some reference to the speech production lexicon during grapheme-phoneme translation. In the experiment varying lexical environment the frequency of responses making use of major correspondences was very low (less than 3 per cent). The structural analysis of the errors indicated that mistakes were more frequent on complex than on simple clusters and that complex vowels were less accurately translated than complex consonants. The errors were in good correspondence with their targets (average similarity = 70 per cent) and consisted mainly of visual confusions and minor translation failures (e.g. boulder → 'builder', canoe → 'canon', bough → 'brought', scene →

TABLE 8.5   *Reaction times (ms) and error rates for lexical and semantic decisions by JM*

			Lexical decisions		
	HF words	LF words	Legal non-words	Illegal non-words	All
X	967	1396[2]	2174[2]	1053	1224
sd	271	712	893	663	723
Error %	7.89	9.09	35[3]	0	10
Rate (ms/letter)		−5	−26	−25	−12

[1] Significant linear trend
[2] Significant effect on reaction time
[3] Significant effect on error rate

'scheme'). There were two phonetic regularisations (heir → 'hair', aisle → 'asel') and two derivational errors (limit → 'limited', eighth → 'eight'). There were no consistent effects on error latencies and no clear tendency for response lexicality to covary with target lexicality or for word error responses to predominate over non-word error responses.

These results suggest that JM read via co-operating morphemic and grapheme-phoneme channels. Route 'g' appears to have functioned on the basis of simple correspondences.

Table 8.5 gives a summary of the results for the semantic and lexical decision tasks. Semantic decisions were made with a slightly elevated error rate and with a reaction time which was high for negative instances and atypical positives. The distribution of RTs had a mean above 2100 ms and was widely dispersed with a tail of slow responses. The typicality effect on positive RT was over 1200 ms. Some inefficiency in the operation of route 'm' to semantics seems to be indicated.

Lexical decision performance was more efficient, with a 10 per cent error rate and a reaction time of 1200 ms overall. The preponderance of reaction times fell below 1250 ms but there was a substantial tail of slower responses, chiefly contributed by the legal non-words. There were large legality effects on both error rate and reaction time and a 400 ms effect of word frequency on positive RT.

The legality effect suggests that JM had successfully internalised orthographic information within the visual processor. This is supported by the results from the array matching task, which show a legality effect of over 300 ms on positive decisions. The data from the visual matching experiments, summarised in Table 8.6, are not in general suggestive of a visual processor impairment. Identity judgments were performed with reaction times and error rates which were well within the normal range. The displays were processed in parallel (except for the vertical format, where the processing rate was 30 ms/letter). Reaction times for array

Typical positives	Atypical positives	Semantic decisions Related negatives	Unrelated negatives	All
1411	2638[2]	2534	2082	2126
654	1689	968	1248	1269
10	25	20[3]	3.45	14.53
				263[1]

matching were also within the normal range, the only noteworthy features being the high error rate on the experiment using mirror image letters and the indications of serial processing in the experiment varying display format.

TABLE 8.6   *Reaction times (ms) and error rates for visual matching tasks by JM*

Experiment		Identity matching		Array matching	
		Overall	Rate (ms/letter)	Overall	Position of difference (ms/position)
1	$\bar{X}$	739	10	$\bar{X}$	1388	36
	sd	191		sd	375	
	Error %	2.5		Error %	10	
2	$\bar{X}$	842	11[1]	$\bar{X}$	1956	231[1]
	sd	181		sd	741	
	Error %	3.09		Error %	20	
3	$\bar{X}$	696	−2	$\bar{X}$	1125	60
	sd	187		sd	396	
	Error %	1.67		Error %	22.97	

[1] Linear trend significant at $p < 0.05$ or better by F-test

The analyses of length effects, summarised in Tables 8.3 and 8.5, gave some evidence of serial processing. This did not apply to lexical decisions which were apparently made by a parallel process. However, the rate for semantic decisions was somewhat above the normal range (260 ms/letter) and the rate for non-word reading was extremely slow (474 ms/letter). Thus, it seems that one element contributing to the delays in JM's non-word reading was a reliance on a slow serial procedure. In word reading, an analysis based on the full distribution of reaction times suggested a rate of about 190 ms/letter. If outliers >3000 ms are removed, this estimate reduces to 90 ms/letter. This is above the range for the competent readers but faster than the rates of the cases considered in the last chapter.

These results suggest the possibility of some impairment to the wholistic function of JM's visual processor. The format distortion results, shown in Table 8.7, also appear indicative of a visual processor disturbance. In all cases other than the semantic decision task the processing rates for the distorted displays were extremely slow. This was particularly true of responses to non-words.

3 Conclusions

JM's Level I description identifies him as a person of average or above average ability whose educational attainment has been limited as a

TABLE 8.7   *Reaction times (ms) and error rates for reading normal and distorted words or non-words by JM*

| | | Vocalisation tasks | | Decision tasks | |
		Words	Non-words	Semantic	Lexical
Normal	X̄	1662	4169	1458	1849
	sd	1456	3661	517	1465
Error %		6.67	36.67	12.5	13.33
	Rate	407[1]	125	91	133
Zigzag	X̄	2126	2971	1888[2]	2496[2]
	sd	1295	1181	919	1786
Error %		3.33	33.33	8.33	13.33
	Rate	298	560[1]	268[1]	199
Vertical	X̄	2375[2]	4423	1843[2]	2658[2]
	sd	1347	2270	617	1669
Error %		10	46.67	10.64	18.33
	Rate	555[1]	972[1]	111	442[1]

[1] Significant linear trend
[2] Format effect on reaction time
[3] Format effect on accuracy

consequence of problems in acquiring basic literacy skills. The possibility of some accompanying language difficulties and visual problems is suggested.

The Level II description, summarised in Table 8.8, is indicative of a multiple impairment in which the major effect is on route 'g' to phonology. Grapheme-phoneme translation involved a very slow serial procedure, vulnerable to disruption by format distortion, operating on simple correspondences with some assistance from stored vocabulary. There were accompanying but relatively milder effects on the morphemic routes to phonology and semantics. Contrary to the standard account of phonological dyslexia, JM made use of the impaired grapheme-phoneme channel when

TABLE 8.8   *Summary of cognitive description of reading functions of subject JM*

Function	Status	Comment
'm' → phonology	Impaired	Frequency effect. Effects of abstract meaning and regularity. Fast serial processing
'g' → phonology	Impaired	Lexicalisation. Difficulty with complex vowels. Slow serial processing
'm' → semantics	Mildly impaired	Large typicality effect. Word frequency effect. Serial processing in semantic decision task
Visual processor	Impaired?	Orthographic model. Slow format resolution. Some serial processing

reading words although there was also evidence of semantic back-up processing. The visual processor functioned normally in tasks involving global or analytic matching but appeared to be open to disruption by distortion and restricted to a serial processing procedure.

Case IV.2   Stephen E (born June 1960)

1   Psycho-educational background

Stephen E was aged 21 years at the start of the research project. His mother reported that he had been born at home and that he had had almost died due to strangulation by the cord and lack of oxygen. Early developmental milestones were considered to have been normally attained, although his mother commented on clumsiness and poor co-ordination. At primary school he had difficulties with number work and spelling, and, to a lesser extent, with reading. His mother reported that he was unhappy at school and was frequently bullied. Some remedial help was given but this was not thought to have been effective. At secondary school Stephen was generally placed with groups of children of low intelligence. He was allowed concessions (use of a tape recorder and, subsequently, a scribe) for his 'O' Grade examinations and passed six subjects at two sittings (English, History, Biology, Chemistry, Metalwork and Engineering Drawing). After leaving school he served an apprenticeship on a farm and took City and Guilds courses in farm and business management. He passed this course (with the concession that his scripts should be typed out after he had written them) and obtained distinctions. He undertook a further course on farm management at an Agricultural College but had difficulty with the work and with note taking. He was allowed no examination concessions and ended by failing the course overall. Since then he has taken a number of different jobs, such as landscape gardening and tractor driving, and, more recently, as a groundsman and storeman on a military base. He attended adult literacy classes on his own initiative when he was 19 years old but the teacher did not feel able to cope with his difficulties in a group situation. Individual tuition was eventually arranged when he was 23 years old. At the age of 20 years a mild epileptic condition was diagnosed. This was treated for two years and the symptoms have now disappeared. He lists his hobbies as reading, listening to music and walking.

An intellectual assessment was carried out in 1984 using the WAIS. The scaled scores are shown in Table 8.9. These are indicative of above average intelligence which is somewhat higher on the verbal scales than on the performance scales. The psychologist noted the difficulty with the digit-symbol test and commented that this was often associated with handwriting problems.

Table 8.10 gives the results from various reading tests which were

TABLE 8.9 *Results of the administration of the WAIS to subject SE (a) in 1981 when subject's CA was 21-7 years and (b) in 1984 when subject's CA was 24-5 years*

	Verbal tests		Performance tests	
a	Similarities	12	Block design	11
	Vocabulary	12	Object assembly	9
	Digit span	10		
	Verbal IQ	108	Performance IQ	99
b	Information	9	Digit symbol	8
	Comprehension	16	Picture completion	11
	Arithmetic	10	Block design	12
	Similarities	13	Picture arrangement	12
	Digit span	11	Object assembly	10
	Vocabulary	13		
	Verbal IQ	112	Performance IQ	103

TABLE 8.10 *Results of administration of reading and spelling tests to subject SE (a) in 1981 when subject's CA was 21-7 years, and (b) in 1984 when subject's CA was 24-5 years*

	Reading ages	Spelling ages
a	Schonell	Schonell
	12-6 years	7-11 years
b	Schonell (test A)	Schonell (test A)
	13-0 years	7-11 years
	Daniels and Diack (test 12)	
	14+ years	
	Schonell (R4 test)	
	13-9 years	

administered in 1981 and 1984. Performance on the graded word lists revealed an ability to read many difficult and unusual words although there were errors due to confusions over letter ordering. Comprehension was good, especially on the untimed test. Nonsense syllable reading was found to be impaired (12/22 correct), suggesting difficulties with phonological assembly.

Testing of spelling was undertaken by means of the Schonell Graded Word test in 1981 and 1984. SE's spelling age was 7-11 years on both occasions, indicating a very severe and persistent impairment. Errors involved b/d confusions and showed a poor grasp of conventional orthographic structure particularly affecting vowel spellings and endings. SE reported that individual help from his tutor had improved his spelling and developed his sense of whether or not a word 'looked right'. In a free writing test he produced an account of his experience of dyslexia which was very well expressed but which included numerous spelling errors and inconsistencies with a lack of punctuation and omission of details such as the crossing of the letter 't'.

SE reported that he had difficulty in distinguishing speech sounds against noisy backgrounds. His general practitioner had tested his hearing by whisper tests on a number of occasions but no formal audiometric assessment had been undertaken. A family history of deafness on his mother's side was mentioned. He scored 82/100 on the Lindamood Auditory Conceptualisation test. The psychologist commented that the level of error was predictive of reading and spelling difficulties in a Primary 5 child and suggested an impaired ability to reflect on and compare the number, identity and sequence of sounds in words.

Orthoptics testing in 1984 established that SE's right eye was fixed as his dominant reference eye and that his vision was normal. No impairment of visual memory for shapes was revealed by an administration of the Graham Kendall test. His results on the Bangor test were within the normal range. Nonetheless, he reported that it was only recently that he had mastered the sequence of the months of the year.

2   Experimental data

A summary of SE's results for reading high frequency words, low frequency words and non-words is given in Table 8.11. The reaction time distributions are displayed in Figure 8.2. SE's reading was accurate, with error levels at about the upper limit of the range for the competent 11 year old readers, although the reaction time levels were clearly elevated.

TABLE 8.11   *Vocal reaction times (ms) and error rates for reading high frequency words, low frequency words and non-words by SE*

| | High frequency words | | | Low frequency words | | | Non-words | | |
	Overall	Intercept	Slope	Overall	Intercept	Slope	Overall	Intercept	Slope
X̄	1466	−259	362[1]	1887	950	199	2903	884	413[1]
sd	1805			1664			1889		
Error %	4.76			11.11			14.83		

[1] Linear trend significant at p<0.05 or better by F-test
Frequency effect t(270) = 1.947, p<0.05. $\chi^2(1)$ = 4.193, p<0.05
Lexicality effect (HF v NW):t(359) = 7.302, p<0.001. $\chi^2(1)$ = 10.461, p<0.001
         (LF v NW):t(311) = 4.74, p<0.001. $\chi^2(1)$ = 0.971

The presence of a 'morphemic dyslexia' is suggested by the inclusion of some slow responses in the distributions for both high and low frequency words. The frequency effect was also somewhat exaggerated (over 400 ms) mainly due to a difference in the number of slow responses in the two

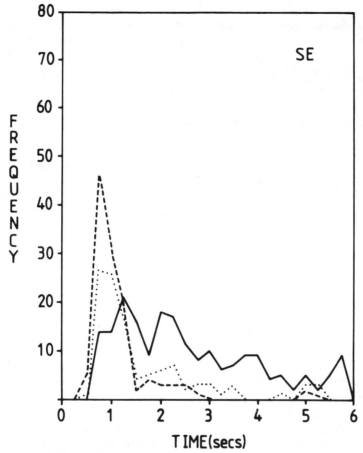

FIGURE 8.2   *Reaction time distributions for responses to high frequency words (– – –), low frequency words (. . .) and non-words (———) by SE*

distributions (18 for high frequency words versus 37 for low frequency words). A more marked 'phonological dyslexia' is indicated by the elevated reaction time for non-word reading (over 2900 ms) and by the dispersed, almost rectangular appearance of the distribution. However, if the error rate of 15 per cent in non-word reading is considered to be within the normal range, SE can be said to exhibit a phonological effect on processing time but not on accuracy.

The analysis of the psycholinguistic variables showed no effects due to the syntactic or semantic factors. Spelling-to-sound irregularity, on the other hand, impaired low frequency word reading. The results, summarised in Table 8.12, show an effect of over 600 ms on reaction time and an increase in error rate from 3 per cent to 39 per cent. These results suggest that SE used his impaired grapheme-phoneme translation channel to support low frequency word reading but that there was no involvement of the semantic processor. The error set included a small number of regularisations (corps → 'corpse', ski → 'sky', ache pronounced as 'H') but these responses were rare and some irregular words which were often regularised by other subjects produced visual confusion errors (canoe → 'canon', sew → 'saw', heir → 'ire', laugh → 'lounge').

TABLE 8.12   *Reaction times (ms) and error rates for reading regular and irregular words of high and low frequency by SE*

| | High frequency words | | Low frequency words | |
	Regular	Irregular	Regular	Irregular
$\overline{X}$	1236	1169	1229	1850[1]
sd	519	488	445	1181
Error %	7.14	10.71	3.57	39.29[2]

[1] Significant effect on reaction time
[2] Significant effect on accuracy

This evidence of lexicalisation in reading was supported by the occurrence of homophony effects on responses to non-words. Homophony reduced the reaction time from over 3000 ms to about 2400 ms (p<0.05). Vowel complexity was associated with a 15 per cent increase in error rate (p<0.05). This difficulty with complex vowels was confirmed by the structural analysis of SE's error set. Only 6 per cent of complex vowels were correctly translated as against over 70 per cent of simple consonants. The analysis of the effects of lexical environment on non-word reading indicated that the use of major correspondences occurred very infrequently (about 6 per cent overall), chiefly as a result of applications of the initial /w/ rule.

Further evidence of a lexical bias comes from a consideration of the frequencies of word and non-word error responses. These data appear in

TABLE 8.14   *Reaction time (ms) and error data for lexical and semantic decisions by SE*

| | | | Lexical decisions | | |
	HF words	LF words	Legal non-words	Illegal non-words	All
$\overline{X}$	2224	2548	3785	3548	2971
sd	1869	1320	1649	2312	2037
Error %	5.26	13.64	20	5	9.17
Rate (ms/letter)		59	1060[1]	865[1]	512[1]

[1] Significant linear trend
[2] Significant effect on reaction time
[3] Significant effect on error rate

Table 8.13 together with the latencies of the error responses. It can be seen that word responses predominated irrespective of the lexicality of the target. The lexical bias was significant by a chi-square test (p<0.01). The error latencies show a large difference between the word → word and non-word → non-word responses (p<0.01). This could reflect the different operational speeds of the 'm' and 'g' routes. It seems clear that SE was extremely reluctant to produce non-word responses to word targets as these were both few in number and had very high latencies (over 14,000 ms).

TABLE 8.13 *Frequencies and latencies (ms) of error responses to word and non-word targets for SE*

	Word		Non-word	
	Word	Non-word	Word	Non-word
$\overline{\text{X}}$	2038	14576	4549	3567
Sd	1025	9182	4180	1864
N	17	6	22	12

The results from the lexical and semantic decision experiments appear in Table 8.14. Semantic decisions were extremely accurate but the reaction time level was elevated, especially for the negative instances, and the distribution was dispersed and included a tail of very slow responses. The distribution has been plotted in Figure 8.3. There was a 550 ms effect of typicality on positive RT. The exaggeration of this effect together with the overall slowness of response suggests some impairment to route 'm' to semantics.

The lexical decision data also give evidence of processing delays. Responses were relatively accurate (9 per cent of errors) but the reaction time was over 2900 ms and the distribution, displayed in Figure 8.3, contained numerous slow responses. SE did not show consistent effects of

	Semantic decisions			
Typical positives	Atypical positives	Related negatives	Unrelated negatives	All
1392	1951[2]	2494	2855	2183
479	853	1399	1947	1419
3.45	0	6.67[3]	0	2.54
				179[1]

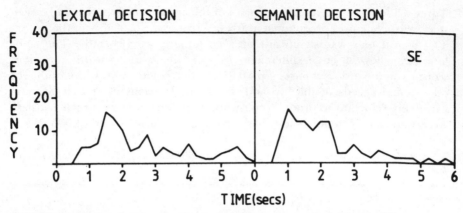

FIGURE 8.3   *Reaction time distributions for lexical and semantic decisions by SE*

frequency on positive responses to words. Negative responses were extremely slow with the RT well above 3000 ms and did not show the usual differentiation between orthographically legal and illegal non-words.

This lack of a legality effect has been illustrated in Figure 8.4 which shows the results from the lexical decision experiment plotted as a function of word and non-word length. The length effects were quite slight for responses to words but very large for both the legal and the illegal non-words. It seems that SE handled these items by an extremely slow serial procedure and that he was unable to make use of information about

TABLE 8.15   *Reaction times (ms) and error rates for reading normal and distorted words or non-words by SE*

		Vocalisation tasks		Decision tasks	
		Words	Non-words	Semantic	Lexical
Normal	$\bar{X}$	1599	3160	1511	2894
	sd	1327	2110	640	1606
Error %		3.33	10	0	5
	Rate	399[1]	393	106	395[1]
Zigzag	$\bar{X}$	2392[2]	4886[2]	2286[2]	3086
	sd	1174	2993	1229	1374
Error %		0	30	4.26	6.67
	Rate	144	820	218	347[1]
Vertical	$\bar{X}$	2027	3736	2469[2]	3352
	sd	743	2162	1568	1568
Error %		6.67	23.33	2.08	11.67
	Rate	302[1]	677[1]	530[1]	508[1]

[1] Significant linear trend
[2] Format effect on reaction time
[3] Format effect on accuracy

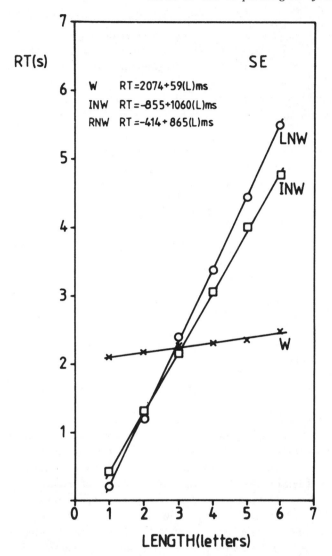

FIGURE 8.4   *Relationship between reaction time word or non-word length in the lexical decision task by subject SE*

orthographic structure to curtail this process in the case of the illegal items.

A tendency towards slow serial processing was also evident in the vocalisation experiments. Following removal of the outliers, the function relating VRT to word length was: $VRT = 560 + 150(L)$ ms. The linear trend test was highly significant. The processing rate in non-word reading was also very slow at over 400 ms/letter. These effects were less clear in the decision tasks. The rate for semantic decisions was 179 ms/letter, which is not greatly outside the range of the competent readers, and there was no significant effect of length on positive lexical decisions.

The format distortion results, which are shown in Table 8.15, are also suggestive of some visual processor inefficiencies. The rates for reading vertically distorted words in the vocalisation and semantic or lexical decision tasks were in the range 400-500 ms/letter and these effects were further exaggerated when responses to non-words were required.

TABLE 8.16   *Reaction times (ms) and error rates for visual matching tasks by SE*

Experiment		Identity matching		Array matching	
		Overall	Rate (ms/letter)	Overall	Position of difference (ms/position)
1	X̄	857	27[1]	X̄	1912	166[1]
	sd	205		sd	639	
	Error %	0.83		Error %	3	
2	X̄	902	26[1]	X̄	2169	210[1]
	sd	280		sd	579	
	Error %	1.85		Error %	5.83	
3	X̄	942	9	X̄	2548	359[1]
	sd	220		sd	791	
	Error %	0		Error %	0.63	

[1] Linear trend significant at $p < 0.05$ or better by F-test

These results suggest a visual processor impairment affecting both the capability for wholistic processing and the application of the procedures necessary to resolve the distortions. Some additional information can be obtained from the visual matching tasks which have been summarised in Table 8.16. Identity matching appears to have been efficiently carried out with very few errors and a reaction time within the normal range. Processing rates were slightly slow at 27 ms/letter in the standard experiment and 47 ms/letter for responses to vertical displays. Array matching was also accurately carried out but the reaction times were at about the level thought to indicate a mild impairment. All three studies gave evidence of serial processing. Contrary to the findings from the lexical decision experiment, there was a significant effect of orthographic legality on the positive RT.

3   Conclusions

SE's Level I description suggests that he is a young man of average or above average intelligence whose educational progress has been disrupted by a severe problem in acquiring spelling competence. The possibility of accompanying language problems is also indicated.

The Level II description is suggestive of a complex pattern of multiple impairments. The summary of the conclusions, contained in Table 8.17, indicates that there were effects on speed of processing in each of the domains. SE possessed an effective grapheme-phoneme convertor which operated by a slow serial procedure on lower level correspondences with some lexical support but with inaccuracies in vowel translation. The morphemic route to phonology also relied on a serial procedure and was somewhat dependent on support from the grapheme-phoneme channel. Nonetheless, word responses predominated within SE's error set. There was also evidence of an effect on speed of processing within the morphemic route to semantics. SE's visual processor appeared to be impaired in its capability for wholistic processing and format resolution. Although orthographic information had been internalised, this was not used to speed rejection of illegal items in the lexical decision task.

TABLE 8.17 *Summary of cognitive description of reading functions of subject SE*

Function	Status	Comment
'm' → phonology	Impaired reaction time	Large frequency effect Grapheme-phoneme support for low frequency words. Bias towards word errors. Slow serial processing
'g' → phonology	Impaired reaction time	Lexical support. Difficulty with complex vowels. Slow serial processing
'm' → semantics	Impaired reaction time	Large typicality effect. No effect of legality on reaction time
Visual processor	Impaired wholistic function	Serial processing. Slow format resolution. Legality effect on matching

Case IV.3 Martin P (born April 1959)

1   Psycho-educational background

Martin was born normally after a long labour 16 days overdue. No family history of learning disabilities was reported. Developmental milestones were stated to have been normally attained. His early schooling was disrupted by family moves and five different primary schools in England and Scotland were attended. One of these moves involved a change from the initial teaching alphabet (ITA) to a standard alphabet. Martin's parents suspected learning difficulties from the age of 5 years onwards. He received remedial teaching in his last year at primary school and throughout his time at seconary school. Following referral to the Tayside Dyslexia Association at the age of about 20 years he undertook a course of individual tuition in reading and spelling. His teacher commented that he appeared to be gaining in confidence and that progress was being made using a phonics-oriented approach. Martin attended a horticultural course at an Agricultural College but was not able to obtain a qualification. He has worked as a general labourer in a factory and as a gardener. He is described as shy and as being largely dependent on his family for social and emotional support. He does not read for pleasure. His hobbies are driving, gardening, swimming and badminton.

Martin's general intelligence was assessed in 1982 by administration of an abbreviated version of the WAIS. This suggested a relatively low level of ability, with Verbal IQ = 85 and Performance IQ = 64. Testing with all sub-tests of the WAIS in 1984 gave the results listed in Table 8.18. These confirm that his intelligence was below average. The scales which appear particularly depressed are oral arithmetic and object assembly. The psychologist commented that low object assembly scores are often associated with poor performance on the Lindamood Auditory Conceptualisation test and that this was the case for MP.

TABLE 8.18 *Results of the administration of the WAIS to subject MP in 1984*

Verbal tests		Performance tests	
Information	8	Digit symbol	5
Comprehension	6	Picture completion	6
Arithmetic	4	Block design	6
Similarities	9	Picture arrangement	8
Digit span	6	Object assembly	4
Vocabulary	8		
Verbal IQ	80	Performance IQ	73

When assessed on behalf of the Association in 1978 Martin was judged on the basis of various tests to have a reading age somewhat above 10 years. An administration of the Schonell graded word test in 1981 gave an age score of 11-8 years. This had remained virtually unaltered when he was reassessed in 1984. Scores on comprehension tests were 13-1 years for the Daniels and Diack untimed test and 10-1 years for the Schonell timed test. MP read 12/22 nonsense words correctly.

A comment from 1978 was that MP's spelling showed an over-dependence on the phonic aspects of words. In 1981 his score on the Schonell graded word test was 10-8 years. This remained much the same when he was retested in 1984. His errors were classed as phonetically plausible attempts with confusions over unstressed vowels. His writing was described as neat with weak spelling and punctuation, inappropriate capitalisation and repetitive expression. Some letters were incorrectly formed.

The 1978 report commented on MP's poor auditory sequential memory (digit span). As noted above, he also performed poorly on the Lindamood Auditory Conceptualisation test in 1984 (51/100). The psychologist commented that this score was predictive of difficulty at the Primary 2 level and was suggestive of a severe defect in the ability to operate on sounds within words. Visual sequential memory was also described as weak in 1978. This was confirmed in 1984 by an administration of the Kendall Memory for Designs test. MP was above the age norms for this test, but, if he is treated as being aged 15-11 years, his difference score is 9, which places him in the 'brain damage' category. MP also had difficulties with the items from the Bangor Dyslexia test. His score was 6, which was regarded as being significant. He had problems with left-right discrimination, repetition of polysyllables, the multiplication tables and the digit span test.

2 Experimental data

Table 8.19 summarises MP's results for the reading of high frequency words, low frequency words and non-words. The reaction time distributions are displayed in Figure 8.5. MP's reading was accurate, with error percentages within or close to the range for the competent 11-year-olds, but very slow. The reaction time distributions for responses to words were widely dispersed and included a tail of very slow responses. The frequency effect was over 1100 ms. The mean response time for non-word reading was over 3400 ms, and the distribution was unusual in shape, being symmetrical in form and centred over the 3000 ms point on the reaction time scale. These data are indicative of a combined morphemic and phonological effect on processing time. The lexicality effect (the difference between non-words and low frequency words) was over 750 ms.

TABLE 8.19 *Vocal reaction times (ms) and error rates for reading high frequency words, low frequency words and non-words by MP*

| | High frequency words | | | Low frequency words | | | Non-words | | |
	Overall	Intercept	Slope	Overall	Intercept	Slope	Overall	Intercept	Slope
X̄	1594	622	196[1]	2696	624	445[1]	3453	1797	340[1]
sd	962			1729			1434		
Error %	2.98			11.9			17.37		

[1] Linear trend significant at $p<0.05$ or better by F-test
Frequency effect: $t(272) = 6.719$, $p<0.001$. $\chi^2(1) = 9.053$, $p<0.01$
Lexicality effect (HF v NW): $t(356) = 14.06$, $p<0.001$. $\chi^2(1) = 20.16$, $p<0.001$
(LF v NW): $t(304) = 4.099$, $p<0.001$. $\chi^2(1) = 1.878$

The analysis of the psycholinguistic effects revealed no influence of form class or abstract versus concrete meaning. Spelling-to-sound irregularity, on the other hand, increased reaction time to high frequency words by 380 ms

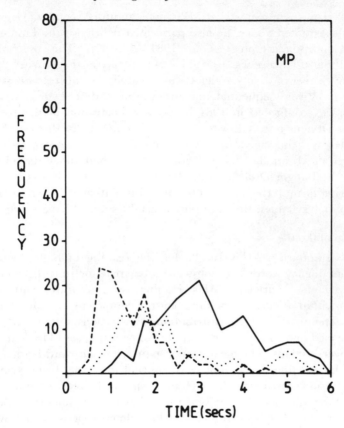

FIGURE 8.5   *Reaction time distributions for responses to high frequency words (– – –), low frequency words (. . .) and non-words (———) by MP*

TABLE 8.21   *Reaction time (ms) and error data for lexical and semantic decisions by MP*

	HF words	LF words	Lexical decisions Legal non-words	Illegal non-words	All
X̄	1014	1528[2]	1849	1398	1320
sd	536	569	1004	757	734
Error %	0	22.73[3]	50[3]	10	15.83
Rate (ms/letter)	187[1]		420	108	177[1]

[1] Significant linear trend
[2] Significant effect on reaction time
[3] Significant effect on error rate

(p<0.01) and raised error rate from 3.57 per cent to 25 per cent (p<0.05). These regularity effects suggest the involvement of some non-lexical phonological processing during word reading (see Table 8.20).

TABLE 8.20   *Reaction times (ms) and error rates for reading regular and irregular words of high and low frequency by MP*

| | High frequency words | | Low frequency words | |
	Regular	Irregular	Regular	Irregular
$\bar{\mathrm{X}}$	1391	1772[1]	2308	2738
sd	588	937	1235	2004
Error %	3.57	7.14	3.57	25[2]

1 Significant effect on reaction time
2 Significant effect on accuracy

In the non-word reading experiment homophony reduced error rate from 25 per cent to 5 per cent (p<0.01). About 11 per cent of responses gave evidence of the use of V+C correspondences, but this tendency was not marked, and only about 14 per cent of items from the consistently irregular set were lexicalised. The structural analysis of errors showed that the responses were in good correspondence with their targets (average similarity = 71 per cent) and that translation errors tended to focus on the complex vowel clusters. These results suggest that MP's translation channel operated on lower level correspondences with some support from the speech production lexicon.

The results from the lexical and semantic decision tasks are shown in Table 8.21. Semantic decisions were accurate for typical positives and unrelated negatives but there were high rates of error for the more difficult atypical positives and related negatives. The reaction time was at about the upper limit of the normal range although the distribution included a tail of

| | Semantic decisions | | | |
Typical positives	Atypical positives	Related negatives	Unrelated negatives	All
1294	1520	2226[2]	1696	1641
651	651	979	643	793
0	26.67[3]	34.48[3]	3.33	16.1
				116[1]

slow responses. The impression that route 'm' to semantics operated efficiently is strengthened by the data from the lexical decision experiment. Performance was accurate and relatively fast for high frequency words and illegal non-words but some delays and errors occurred in the responses to lower frequency words and legal non-words. The reaction time distribution was again well formed although it included a tail of slower responses.

The legality effects on lexical decision RT and accuracy suggest that MP had internalised a model of English orthography. This is confirmed by the results from the array matching task, where legal letter arrays were matched about 300 ms faster than illegal arrays ($p<0.05$). However, MP's performance on the matching tasks was in general very slow. The data have been summarised in Table 8.22 which shows results for the identity matching and array matching experiments. Identity matching was accurate but slow in the format distortion version where vertical displays were processed with a rate of 90 ms/letter. In array matching, reaction times were well above the normal range for all three experiments. There was evidence of slow serial processing with a rate of 300-400 ms/position in two of the experiments. These data are suggestive of a generalised inefficiency within MP's visual processor.

TABLE 8.22   *Reaction times (ms) and error rates for visual matching by MP*

| Experiment | | Identity matching | | | Array matching | |
		Overall	Rate (ms/letter)		Overall	Position of difference (ms/position)
1	X̄	961	19[1]	X̄	2613	331[1]
	sd	308		sd	849	
	Error %	0.83		Error %	4	
2	X̄	1453	42[1]	X̄	3142	438[1]
	sd	515		sd	1023	
	Error %	0.62		Error %	5	
3	X̄	1212	−28	X̄	3070	14
	sd	522		sd	891	
	Error %	0		Error %	3.13	

[1] Linear trend significant at $p<0.05$ or better by F-test

The effects of word length, included in Tables 8.19 and 8.20, are indicative of serial processing. If the data for word reading are analysed with outliers >3500 ms removed the obtained processing rates are 163 ms/letter for high frequency words and 148 ms/letter for low frequency words. There is evidence of slow serial processing for responses to words in the lexical decision task and in the reading aloud of non-words

(340 ms/letter), but not in the semantic decision task.

MP's performance was seriously disrupted by the format distortions. The data have been summarised in Table 8.23. Distortion had significant effects on accuracy in the word and non-word reading experiments. The processing rates for reading distorted items were generally very slow, exceeding 300 ms/letter for semantic decisions, 400 ms/letter for lexical decisions, and showing much slower rates for the vocalisation tasks.

TABLE 8.23 *Reaction times (ms) and error rates for reading normal and distorted words or non-words by MP*

		Vocalisation tasks		Decision tasks	
		Words	Non-words	Semantic	Lexical
Normal	$\bar{X}$	1913	2876	1629	1777
	sd	765	1340	820	930
Error %		3.33	6.67	4.17	10
	Rate	222^1	496^1	114	116
Zigzag	$\bar{X}$	2956^2	4588^2	2418^2	2746^2
	sd	1378	2580	1173	1232
Error %		20^3	23.33	10.87	13.33
	Rate	722^1	1001^1	382^1	410^1
Vertical	$\bar{X}$	3922^2	5638^2	2614^2	3001^2
	sd	1935	2530	1141	1429
Error %		13.33	43.33^3	14.58	21.67
	Rate	743^1	845^1	354^1	407^1

[1] Significant linear trend
[2] Format effect on reaction time
[3] Format effect on accuracy

3 Conclusions

MP's Level I description indicates that he is a young man of low general intelligence, especially in the performance area, with a somewhat disrupted educational history, who has attained a modest level of competence in reading and spelling. Quite severe accompanying difficulties in auditory conceptualisation and visual processing are indicated.

The Level II description, summarised in Table 8.24, is suggestive of the presence of a visual processor impairment combined with effects on the speed of operation of routes 'g' and 'm' to phonology. MP's visual processor appeared to operate on a slow serial basis and was inefficient in making analytic visual comparisons and resolving format distortions. Despite this, the morphemic route to semantics functioned relatively efficiently aside from some inaccuracies in classifying marginal instances of categories. The 'm' and 'g' routes to phonology were both impaired with respect to time and relied on a serial process. There was evidence that word retrieval was

TABLE 8.24   *Summary of cognitive description of reading functions of subject MP*

Function	Status	Comment
'm' → phonology	Impaired reaction time	Large frequency effect. Support by grapheme-phoneme translation. Slow serial processing
'g' → phonology	Impaired	Lexical support. Errors on complex vowels. Slow serial processing
'm' → semantics	Efficient?	Inaccurate on atypical items and related negatives. Serial processing in lexical decisions
Visual processor	Impaired	Orthographic model. Very slow array matching. Serial processing. Errors on distorted formats. Slow resolution of zigzag and vertical distortions

aided by grapheme-phoneme translation and that the translation process was supported by reference to the speech production lexicon.

Conclusions: Series IV

The three subjects considered in this series are somewhat heterogeneous and do not conform to a standard view of phonological dyslexia. All three give evidence of an effect on the grapheme-phoneme translation process. However, this was combined with other impairments and did not lead to a commitment to a lexicalised or semantic mode of reading.

Subject JM's Level I description gave indications of language difficulties, reflected particularly in the poor score on the Lindamood test. At Level II, the phonological dyslexia was clearly marked by the reaction time and error rates in non-word reading. There were accompanying effects on the visual processor and on the morphemic routes. Despite the phonological impairment, the grapheme-phoneme channel was used to support word retrieval. The error set did not include a predominance of derivational or semantic errors or of word responses.

Subject SE's phonological dyslexia was indexed primarily by slowness of translation time. He also showed accompanying effects on the 'm' routes and some visual processor anomalies, including an inability to take advantage of orthographic illegalities in the word/non-word discrimination task. At Level I, his predominant feature was an extreme impairment of spelling ability.

MP's results provide a second opportunity to consider the effects of a low level of intelligence on reading performance. His Level I description suggests the presence of widespread impairments affecting visual processing, auditory conceptualisation and other functions. At Level II, he showed processing delays in all systems, although route 'm' to semantics was relatively less affected.

8.3 Series V case studies: severe phonological effect

This section will present details of five further cases in whom the phonological effect was severe. The order of presentation has again been determined by a ranking of efficiency in reading high frequency words.

Case V.1 Stephen B (born April 1968)

1 Psycho-educational background

Stephen, an only child, was born 6 to 7 weeks prematurely but without complications, having been diagnosed as 'hyperkinetic *in utero*'. Developmental milestones were normal although he did not crawl. He injured his head in a fall from a climbing frame at 3-9 years and there was a squint in both eyes for four months following the accident. He had four hospitalisations pre-school, each for 2 or 3 weeks, on account of an allergic reaction to polio and triple vaccine. Learning difficulties were suspected from the age of 7 years and were sympathetically considered by the school authorities. He received additional tuition from the Tayside Dyslexia Association and from his mother, a qualified teacher, and was provided with weekly individual help at secondary school. In 1980 his Association teacher commented that he was progressing well but that his concept of sounds was still poor and she was accordingly concentrating on a phonics approach. A school report from the same period was very positive. Stephen did well at 'O' Grade with band A results in Mathematics, Arithmetic, Physics, Chemistry and Biology and average passes in English and Geography (for which a spelling concession was allowed). He is studying five subjects at the Higher Grade and plans to remain at school for a sixth year and then to go to university to study biophysics. His interests are mainly outdoors (riding, swimming, ski-ing, cycling, golf) but he likes TV and computers and has recently started to read for pleasure. SB is right-handed and right-footed. Both his mother and his mother's niece were reported to have experienced learning difficulties.

Stephen's general intelligence was assessed by administration of an abbreviated WISC in 1979. His scores were above average, especially in the performance area (Verbal IQ = 113, Performance IQ = 132). The full set of scales from the WISC were administered as part of a re-assessment in 1984. The scaled scores have been summarised in Table 8.25 and can be seen to confirm the earlier conclusions. The only areas which show a slight depression are information on the verbal scale and coding on the performance scale. The information errors included confusion about the direction of the setting sun, the number of grams in a kilogram and the identities of the four seasons.

TABLE 8.25   *Results of the administration of the WISC to subject SB (a) in 1979, when subject's CA was 10-11 years, and (b) in 1984 when subject's CA was 16-6 years*

	Verbal tests		Performance tests	
a	Similarities	15	Block design	15
	Vocabulary	11	Object assembly	14
	Digit span	10		
	Verbal IQ	113	Performance IQ	132
b	Information	9	Picture completion	15
	Similarities	11	Picture arrangement	16
	Arithmetic	13	Block design	13
	Vocabulary	11	Object assembly	16
	Comprehension	15	Coding	10
	Digit span	13		
	Verbal IQ	112	Performance IQ	129

TABLE 8.26   *Results of administration of reading and spelling tests to subject SB (a) in 1979 when subject's CA was 10-11 years, (b) in 1981 when subject's CA was 12-9 years, and (c) in 1984 when subject's CA was 16-6 years*

	Reading ages		Spelling ages	
	Neale Analysis		Daniels and Diack	
a	rate	8-5 years		7-7 years
	accuracy	8-9 years		
	comprehension	9-3 years		
	Neale Analysis		Daniels and Diack	
b	rate	11-0 years		8-2 years
	accuracy	8-9 years		
	comprehension	9-6 years		
	Daniels and Diack (test 12)			
		11-6 years		
	Schonell (test A)		Schonell (test A)	
c		12-0 years		11-2 years
	Daniels and Diack (test 12)			
		12-6 years		
	Schonell (R4 test)			
		11-11 years		

Table 8.26 gives a summary of the results of formal tests of SB's reading abilities. These establish that he was impaired in reading speed, accuracy and comprehension throughout the period of investigation. In 1984 the educational psychologist commented that his reading was slow and that there were many minor inaccuracies. He scored only 14/22 on a test of reading nonsense words.

Handwriting was described as legible in 1984 with satisfactory content but occasional omission of full stops and inflections. The results of formal spelling tests are given in Table 8.26 and show a consistent impairment. The psychologist noted the occurrence of sequence errors and uncertainty over consonant doubling and vowel spellings.

SB showed no evidence of a visual memory impairment on the Graham Kendall test. Orthoptics testing indicated that his vision was normal and that his right eye was established as a stable reference eye. Application of the Lindamood Auditory Conceptualisation test in 1984 gave a score of 82/100. The psychologist commented that the difficulty was mainly in the 'manipulation of sequence' and that the score was predictive of difficulties in a child at the Primary 5 level. SB did not give positive results on the Bangor dyslexia test.

2   Experimental data

Table 8.27 gives a summary of the results from the word and non-word reading experiments. The plot of the frequency distributions appears in Figure 8.6. The results are indicative of a combined morphemic and phonological dyslexia, with the phonological effect being relatively the more severe. The 'morphemic dyslexia' is indicated by (1) errors and occasional slow responses when reading high frequency words, (2) numerous errors and slow responses when reading low frequency words, and (3) an exaggeration of the word frequency effect to over 970 ms. The 'phonological dyslexia' is shown by a very high error rate in non-word reading (44 per cent) and a dispersed distribution with a mean over 3000 ms and large numbers of slow responses. The lexicality effect was over 1000 ms.

TABLE 8.27   *Vocal reaction times (ms) and error rates for reading high frequency words, low frequency words and non-words by SB*

	High frequency words			Low frequency words			Non-words		
	Overall	Intercept	Slope	Overall	Intercept	Slope	Overall	Intercept	Slope
X̄	1031	414	131[1]	2008	445	341	3055	−272	707[1]
sd	648			2093			3107		
Error %	16.67			32.54			44.07		

[1] Linear trend significant at p<0.05 or better by F-test
   Frequency effect: $t(223) = 5.109$, $p<0.001$. $\chi^2(1) = 10.1$, $p<0.01$
   Lexicality effect (HF v NW): $t(270) = 7.507$, $p<0.001$. $\chi^2(1) = 33.496$, $p<0.001$
                  (LF v NW): $t(215) = 2.72$, $p<0.005$. $\chi^2(1) = 4.547$, $p<0.02$

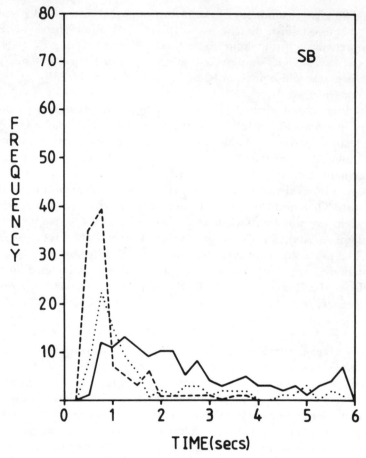

FIGURE 8.6   *Reaction time distributions for responses to high frequency words (– – –), low frequency words (. . .) and non-words (———) by SB*

Speed and accuracy of word reading were not affected by form class but there was an effect of over 1000 ms of abstract meaning on reaction time to read low frequency words ($p<0.025$). This effect is shown in Table 8.28. The large standard deviations associated with the abstract words indicate that these items contributed disproportionately to the production of slow responses by SB. Some involvement of semantic processing in word retrieval is implied. Spelling-to-sound irregularity had no effect on reaction time but raised error rate for reading low frequency words from 14.29 per cent to 46.43 per cent ($p<0.01$). This indicates that, despite the severe phonological dyslexia, SB made use of the grapheme-phoneme translation channel when reading. His error set included three possible regularisations (heir → 'hair, ache → 'arch', concept → 'conkept'), and three derivational errors (these → 'this', know → 'known', eighth → 'eighty').

TABLE 8.28   *Reaction times (ms) and error rates for reading function words and concrete and abstract word of high and low frequency by SB*

| | High frequency words | | | Low frequency words | |
	Function	Concrete	Abstract	Concrete	Abstract
$\bar{X}$	955	823	1239	1040	2062[1]
sd	679	291	1021	347	1487
Error %	9.52	14.29	23.81	28.57	33.33

[1] Significant effect on reaction time
[2] Significant effect on accuracy

SB's non-word reading was affected by vowel complexity and homophony. Homophony reduced error rate from 48 to 28 per cent (p<0.05) and complexity increased error rate by more than 30 per cent (p<0.001) and raised the reaction time by over 700 ms. The effect of vowel complexity was confirmed in the structural analysis of SB's errors. Out of 122 complex vowel groups occurring in his error sample only 16 per cent were correctly translated. Aside from this errors were in reasonable structural correspondence with their targets (average similarity = 62 per cent). Only a small percentage of responses to non-words showed a readiness to make use of major correspondences (16 per cent). These data suggest the availability of an operational channel using primitive correspondences which was very inaccurate in vowel translation.

SB produced both word and non-word errors. Target and response lexicality tended to covary (p<0.01) with about 60 per cent of responses being from the same class as the target. Errors involving word responses to words had much shorter latencies than errors involving non-word responses to non-words (1971 ms versus 4123 ms, p<0.01). This difference parallels the effect observed for correct responses. The latency for word responses to non-words was 2700 ms, suggesting some advantage for lexicalisation of output from the translation channel.

Table 8.29 gives the results from the lexical and semantic decision experiments. SB's performance was characterised by fast responses combined with a high rate of error. The reaction times were well within the normal range but SB made numerous mistakes on atypical positives and related negatives in the semantic decision task and on low frequency words and legal non-words in the lexical decision task.

A general impression given by SB is that he tended systematically to trade accuracy for speed. This was also apparent in the visual matching tasks, summarised in Table 8.30. Identity matching was performed with a reaction time which was below the range for the competent readers although the error rates on two of the experiments were elevated. The standard array matching experiment also involved very fast reactions combined with a 25 per cent error rate, attributable particularly to mistakes

TABLE 8.29   *Reaction time (ms) and error data for lexical and semantic decisions by SB*

		HF words	LF words	Lexical decisions Legal non-words	Illegal non-words	All
	$\bar{X}$	708	791	822	788	765
	sd	143	200	203	131	163
Error %		13.16	27.27	45^3	7.5	19.17
Rate (ms/letter)			27	68	2	21

[1] Significant linear trend
[2] Significant effect on reaction time
[3] Significant effect on error rate

TABLE 8.30   *Reaction times (ms) and error rates for visual matching by SB*

Experiment		Identity matching Overall	Rate (ms/letter)		Array matching Overall	Position of difference (ms/position)
1	$\bar{X}$	573	4	$\bar{X}$	778	−2
	sd	104		sd	238	
	Error %	13.33		Error %	25	
2	$\bar{X}$	593	10^1	$\bar{X}$	1112	121^1
	sd	145		sd	335	
	Error %	11.11		Error %	11.67	
3	$\bar{X}$	534	-6^1	$\bar{X}$	912	36
	sd	81		sd	269	
	Error %	5		Error %	13.75	

[1] Linear trend significant at $p<0.05$ or better by F-test

on mismatching items. There was no legality effect and no evidence of serial processing except in the experiment varying horizontal and vertical format.

According to this interpretation, the functions of the visual processor and route 'm' to phonology might be considered to be efficient apart from a liability to error due to a tendency to curtail processing too early to allow more difficult discriminations to be made. The analysis of length and format effects was also suggestive of efficient visual processing. There were no significant length effects in the lexical decision experiment. The rate for semantic decisions, following removal of two outliers, was only 70 ms/letter. Rates were somewhat higher in the word vocalisation experiments but reduced to 65 ms/letter when the outlying responses were disregarded. This rate is somewhat slower than that of the competent readers but not greatly so. As is to be expected in phonological dyslexia, the rate for non-word reading was extremely slow (over 700 ms/letter).

Typical positives	Semantic decisions			All
	Atypical positives	Related negatives	Unrelated negatives	
682	864	1095	1419	1012
494	459	593	1365	900
10	37.93[3]	41.38[3]	16.67	26.27
				71[1]

Table 8.31 shows the effects of the format distortions. The impact of this variation was relatively slight in the lexical and semantic decision experiments. Much slower processing occurred in the vocalisation tasks but this seems to have been true for normal and distorted displays alike.

TABLE 8.31 *Reaction times (ms) and error rates for reading normal and distorted words or non-words by SB*

| | | Vocalisation tasks | | Decision tasks | |
		Words	Non-words	Semantic	Lexical
Normal	$\bar{\text{X}}$	1693	2447	736	880
	sd	1658	1561	336	350
Error %		10	26.67	20.83	26.67
Rate		431[1]	513[1]	−1	76[1]
Zigzag	$\bar{\text{X}}$	1989	2601	752	927
	sd	1491	1504	248	447
Error %		13.33	40	21.28	31.67
Rate		248	453[1]	−1	73
Vertical	$\bar{\text{X}}$	1894	3158	951[2]	1073[2]
	sd	1097	1640	394	616
Error %		10	40	17.02	43.33
Rate		408[1]	574[1]	112[1]	77

[1] Significant linear trend
[2] Format effect on reaction time
[3] Format effect on accuracy

3 Conclusions

SB's Level I description identifies him as a boy of above average intelligence, especially in the non-verbal area, who is strongly motivated to succeed academically despite a disability affecting reading and spelling.

His Level II description, summarised in Table 8.32, indicates the presence of a severe phonological dyslexia combined with a morphemic dyslexia. There is evidence of interaction between the 'g' and 'm' routes. The visual processor and route 'm' to semantics appear efficient aside from the strategic bias in favour of trading accuracy for speed.

TABLE 8.32   *Summary of cognitive description of reading functions of subject SB*

Function	Status	Comment
'm' → phonology	Impaired	Large frequency effect. Support by semantic processing. Support by grapheme-phoneme processing
'g' → phonology	Very impaired	Lexical support. Difficulty with complex vowels. Slow serial processing
'm' → semantics	Efficient	Trades accuracy for speed
Visual processor	Efficient	Trades accuracy for speed

Case V.S   Laura T (born October 1962)

1   Psycho-educational background

Laura is the fourth of four children and was born, unattended, on a hospital trolley at full term following a short labour. She reported that her mother and older sister had experienced reading and spelling difficulties. She was described as a clumsy child. She did not crawl but learned to walk early. No speech or communication difficulties were recorded. She was slow in learning to tie her shoelaces and to read the clock and was confused about left and right. A possible learning disability was suspected before she started school because, unlike other members of the family, she was unable to learn to write her name. She had difficulty with reading at primary school and reported that she used to try to learn the texts by rote at home so that she could recite them without having to read them in school. Her headteacher refused a request for referral to the school psychological service but provided group remedial help together with children of duller intelligence. This proved not to be helpful. When the local Tayside Dyslexia Association was formed an assessment was undertaken and individual tuition was arranged and maintained until the end of her fifth year at secondary school. She passed seven subjects at 'O' Grade and three at the Higher Grade (Chemistry, Mathematics and English) with the concession that she be permitted the help of a scribe in the English examinations. She gained entrance to university and successfully pursued courses leading to admission to the honours class in microbiology. In her university examinations the question papers are read to her. She enjoys sports such as badminton and squash. She is married and has a small daughter.

An assessment of general intelligence was made in 1984 using the WAIS. The scaled sub-test scores, which appear in Table 8.33, are indicative of above average ability in both the verbal and the performance spheres. The psychologist commented on the depression of the digit span and the oral arithmetic scores as presenting a 'typically dyslexic pattern' and noted that her vocabulary score was somewhat reduced by imprecision in her explanations of meaning and the occurrence of some 'dyslexic-type mistakes' such as defining breakfast as 'the first day of the meal'. The depression of picture completion among the performance tests was considered indicative of a poor visual memory, or, more probably, poor figure-ground discrimination.

TABLE 8.33   *Results of the administration of the WAIS to subject LT in 1984*

Verbal tests		Performance tests	
Information	12	Digit symbol	13
Comprehension	17	Picture completion	9
Arithmetic	9	Block design	13
Similarities	14	Picture arrangement	11
Digit span	6	Object assembly	13
Vocabulary	13		
Verbal IQ	111	Performance IQ	111

LT completed a Schonell graded word test in 1981 and obtained a reading age of 11-5 years. Repetition of this test in 1984 gave a score of 12-8 years. On both occasions her errors included derivational paralexias (imagine → 'image', gradually → 'gradual', applaud → 'applause', nourished → 'nutrition') and visual confusions. On the test of reading non-words she scored only 8/22, indicating a serious weakness in phonological assembly. However, her scores on the Daniels and Diack and Schonell tests of comprehension were at ceiling.

LT's spelling age, assessed by the Schonell test, was 11-6 years in 1981 and 11-11 years in 1984. The psychologist commented on the occurrence of b/d reversals, sound/letter mismatch, consonant doubling confusions and omission of sounds and ordering errors. LT's free writing was said to be legible but with incorrect punctuation, b/d reversals, and poor spelling, including mis-spelling of technical terms from her university course.

Laura wears contact lenses but reported no special visual problems. Her performance on the Graham Kendall test did not indicate any impairment of shape memory. There were no reports of hearing problems and her speech was fluent apart from the minor conceptual confusions already mentioned. On the Lindamood test she scored 76/100 which was considered predictive of difficulties at the middle primary level and as indicative of a severe weakness in the ability to reflect on and compare the identity, number and sequence of sounds in words. The psychologist suggested that these difficulties related to both phoneme representation and phoneme segmentation. On the Bangor tests, she obtained a positive score of 6. She had difficulties with repetition of polysyllables, recall of the multiplication tables, and with temporal and spatial concepts.

2   Experimental data

LT's results for reading words of high and low frequency are displayed in Table 8.34. The reaction time distributions appear in Figure 8.7. The data are strongly suggestive of the presence of a 'phonological dyslexia'. This is indicated by the high error rate in non-word reading (31 per cent), by the very slow reaction time for non-word reading (over 3800 ms) and by the dispersed Type C reaction time distribution. Non-word reading was differentiated from low frequency word reading in terms of both accuracy and reaction time. The lexicality effect was over 2000 ms.

TABLE 8.34   *Vocal reaction times (ms) and error rates for reading high frequency words, low frequency words and non-words by LT*

| | High frequency words | | | Low frequency words | | | Non-words | | |
	Overall	Intercept	Slope	Overall	Intercept	Slope	Overall	Intercept	Slope
X̄	1247	315	196[1]	1790	878	193	3858	2469	288[1]
sd	1362			1719			2467		
Error %	7.74			16.67			31.06		

[1] Linear trend significant at p<0.05 or better by F-test
  Frequency effect: t(258) = 2.821, p<0.005. $\chi^2(1)$ = 5.612, p<0.02
  Lexicality effect (HF v NW):t(315) = 11.554, p<0.001, $\chi^2(1)$ = 31.754, p<0.01
               (LF v NW):t(265) = 7.461, p<0.001, $\chi^2(1)$ = 8.828, p<0.01

The data for word reading provide evidence of an accompanying 'morphemic dyslexia'. The error levels were elevated relative to those of the competent 11-year-old readers and slow responses occurred, especially to the lower frequency words.

LT exhibits a combined phonological and morphemic dyslexia in which the phonological effect appears to be the more severe. According to the standard model of phonological dyslexia, this configuration should result in an absence of effects of regularity and an influence of semantic variables on word reading. There were no significant effects of regularity on either reaction time or error rate. The data from the experiment varying abstract versus concrete meaning have been summarised in Table 8.35. Abstract meaning did not affect error rates but did increase the dispersion of the

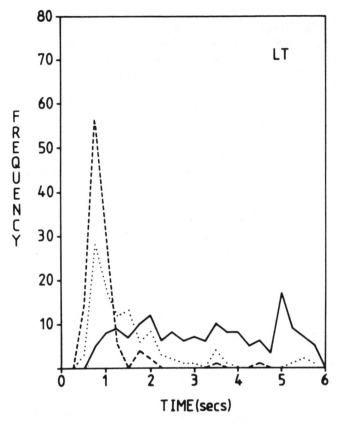

FIGURE 8.7   *Reaction time distributions for responses to high frequency words (– – –), low frequency words (. . .) and non-words (———) by LT*

TABLE 8.35   *Reaction times (ms) and error rates for reading function words and concrete and abstract words of high and low frequency by LT*

| | High frequency words | | | Low frequency words | |
	Function	Concrete	Abstract	Concrete	Abstract
X̄	1799[1]	1032	1149	1274	2285
sd	2426	651	812	444	2909
Error %	2.38	0	9.52	4.76	4.76

[1] Significant effect on reaction time
[2] Significant effect on accuracy

reaction time distributions. There was a clear effect of the function/content distinction on reaction time. The mean RT for function word reading was almost 1800 ms and this was significantly greater than the RT to read other high frequency words. These effects suggest some involvement of syntactic and semantic processing in word retrieval.

LT's non-word reading was affected by homophony which reduced reaction time from over 4000 ms to 2800 ms (p<0.01). This implies that the output from the grapheme-phoneme translator was 'lexicalised' by referral to the vocabulary store. In the experiment varying the lexical environments of non-words only about 9 per cent of responses were lexicalised (e.g. molf pronounced to rhyme with 'wolf', vold → /voold/, quatch → 'quotch', prall → 'prawl', etc). Thus, there was some use of V+C correspondences, though the frequency was relatively low.

A feature of adult phonological dyslexia is an absence of phonetic regularisation errors and the occurrence of some derivational errors. LT made only one error which appeared to involve a regularisation (ought → 'out') but produced four clear derivational errors (variety → 'vary', crept → 'creep', hunger → 'hungry', beauty → 'beautiful'). There were also two visually similar errors which may have involved a semantic component (rhyme → 'rhythm', quest → 'question'). LT also produced a number of visual confusion errors (liberty → 'library', poach → 'pouch', grant → 'grunt').

Table 8.36 gives the frequencies and latencies of word and non-word error responses to word and non-word targets. LT showed a strong tendency for response lexicality and target lexicality to covary (p<0.001 by chi-square test). Word responses to words were also made with a substantially faster latency than non-word responses to non-words (p<0.001). The results are consistent with the proposal that word → word errors were generally produced by the relatively unimpaired morphemic route whereas the other error responses involved the slow operation of route 'g'. Since non-word → word errors have a relatively high latency (over 4100 ms), it seems likely that they were generated by matching of the output from route 'g' against stored vocabulary rather than by a process of confusion within the morphemic input channel.

These results make it clear that LT made use of her impaired grapheme-phoneme channel in reading and that it was involved in the production of the majority of her error responses. The errors involved vowel confusions

TABLE 8.36 *Latencies (ms) and frequencies of word and non-word error responses to word and non-word targets by LT*

	Words		Non-words	
	Words	Non-words	Words	Non-words
X̄	1879	4131	4204	5620
sd	1569	2198	2086	4017
N	28	7	24	48

(deft → 'dift', sproot → 'sprout', brawd → 'browd'), consonant confusions (won → 'mon', glab → 'clab', stimp → 'strimp', paich → 'painch'), and letter ordering errors (gloat → 'goalt', threm → 'therm', dosk → 'doks', frosk → 'forsk'). It can be seen from these examples that the responses were generally in good structural correspondence with their targets. The structural analysis of the errors gave an average similarity score of 66 per cent, wth 91 per cent of errors having a score of 50 per cent or better. The mistranslations tended to focus on the complex clusters, especially the vowels.

The results from the decision experiments were examined with the aim of assessing the state of route 'm' to semantics and of the visual processor. Data from the lexical and semantic decision tasks have been summarised in Table 8.37. Semantic decisions were made rapidly and with a low error rate and fell well within the range for the competent readers. The reaction time distribution was well formed. Results for the lexical decision task were also indicative of efficient processing. The error rate was only 6 per cent overall and reaction times were within a normal range for all items except the legal non-words. If the delay in classification of legal non-words is treated as a consequence of LT's phonological impairment, then it seems reasonable to conclude that route 'm' to semantics operated efficiently.

The analysis of LT's visual processor functions also suggested the absence of an impairment. Performance on the visual matching tasks, summarised in Table 8.38, fell within or below the accuracy and reaction time levels shown by the competent readers. There was some evidence of significant length and position effects in the two tasks but the rates were fast and within the normal range. There was no significant effect of legality on reaction time in the array matching task.

The data on length effects, included in Tables 8.34 and 8.37, are not indicative of serial processing. Positive lexical decisions and semantic decisions showed no consistent word length effects. Rates of processing in the vocalisation tasks were considerably slower. However, if the word data are analysed with outliers >3000 ms removed the length effect reduces to 58 ms/letter. Thus, morphemic access to the phonological system may have involved some serial processing but not the very slow procedure observed in the cases of morphemic dyslexia discussed in the last chapter.

Table 8.39 indicates that LT was also relatively unaffected by the format distortions. In the lexical and semantic decisions experiments distortion had very little impact on either accuracy or reaction time and there was no indication of an interaction with word length. Numerically larger length effects occurred in the vocalisation tasks but they were generally not significant and occurred for normal formats as well as for the distortions.

TABLE 8.37   *Reaction times (ms) and error data for lexical and semantic decisions by LT*

	HF words	LF words	Lexical decisions Legal non-words	Illegal non-words	All
$\bar{\text{X}}$	796	889	2252[2]	859	1083
sd	267	324	1813	361	954
Error %	2.63	9.09	20[3]	0	5.83
Rate (ms/letter)		−6	876[1]	123[1]	150

[1] Significant linear trend
[2] Significant effect on reaction time
[3] Significent effect on error rate

TABLE 8.38   *Reaction times (ms) and error rates for visual matching tasks by LT*

Experiment		Identity matching Overall	Rate (ms/letter)		Array matching Overall	position of difference (ms/position)
1	$\bar{\text{X}}$	543	7[1]	$\bar{\text{X}}$	760	27
	sd	116		sd	180	
	Error %	5		Error %	13	
2	$\bar{\text{X}}$	607	11[1]	$\bar{\text{X}}$	1166	135[1]
	sd	167		sd	389	
	Error %	5.56		Error %	11.67	
3	$\bar{\text{X}}$	514	−6	$\bar{\text{X}}$	1038	−2
	sd	120		sd	427	
	Error %	3.33		Error %	15.63	

[1] Linear trend significant at $p < 0.05$ or better by F-test

3   Conclusions

LT's Level I analysis defines her as a young woman of above average ability who has succeeded academically despite serious dyslexic problems in learning to read and spell. An accompanying difficulty in auditory conceptualisation is suggested.

The Level II description, summarised in Table 8.40, is indicative of a severe and relatively isolated phonological dyslexia. LT's grapheme-phoneme translator was liable to error on complex clusters and processed information extremely slowly. The homophony effect suggested that the output was occasionally 'lexicalised' by matching against stored vocabulary. Nonetheless, it is important to stress that LT's translation channel was operational. This is indicated by the high frequency of non-word

Typical positives	Semantic decisions Atypical positives	Related negatives	Unrelated negatives	All
838	1158	1415	1156	1136
256	1125	716	575	759
3.33	6.9	10	3.45	5.93
				70

TABLE 8.39   *Reaction times (ms) and error rates for reading normal and distorted words or non-words by LT*

		Vocalisation tasks Words	Non-words	Decision tasks Semantic	Lexical
Normal	$\bar{X}$	1307	4483	793	790
	sd	793	2878	254	324
Error	%	6.67	20	6.25	8.33
	Rate	234[1]	339	18	−32
Zigzag	$\bar{X}$	1989	5574	968[2]	1048[2]
	sd	2537	5503	397	658
Error	%	6.67	20	14.89	10
	Rate	427	141	110[1]	−21
Vertical	$\bar{X}$	1625	5872	1020[2]	1068[2]
	sd	789	4607	447	552
Error	%	13.33	33.33	8.51	16.67
	Rate	230[1]	385	64	34

[1] Significant linear trend
[2] Format effect on reaction time
[3] Format effect on accuracy

responses and by the demonstrations that a majority of errors were products of erroneous grapheme-phoneme translation. The process was also relatively accurate. About 70 per cent of non-words were correctly read and errors were generally structurally close to the targets.

The effect on route 'g' was accompanied by a milder effect on route 'm' to phonology. This was indexed by the occurrence of visual confusion errors, derivational errors and delays in reading function words and words of abstract meaning. These syntactic/semantic effects imply some involvement of semantic processing in word retrieval. The absence of a regularity effect or of phonetic regularisation errors suggests that word reading was

TABLE 8.40 *Summary of cognitive description of reading functions of subject LT*

Function	Status	Comment
'm' → phonology	Impaired	Large frequency effect. Function word effect. Derivational errors
'g' → phonology	Very impaired	Lexical support. Difficulty with complex vowels
'm' → semantics	Efficient	Slow rejection of legal non-words
Visual processor	Efficient	

not in general supported by route 'g'. The use of the route may have been restricted to the non-word reading tasks, possibly including negative responses to legal non-words when making lexical decisions.

LT's visual processor appeared to be unimpaired in that she did not give any strong evidence for serial reading, delays in matching, or difficulties in resolving format distortions. The only questionable feature was the absence of a legality effect on performance in the array matching task. This could be taken to imply the absence of an internalised model of English orthography. On the other hand, negative lexical decisions were sensitive to legality, and so it may be that the orthographic information was available even though it was not used.

Route 'm' to semantics appeared to function efficiently. This result is important because it stands as a counter-example to the earlier indications that the two morphemic routes tend to be jointly impaired. LT's data show that route 'm' to semantics may function on the basis of fast parallel processing despite the occurrence of delays and some serial processing and other inefficiencies in route 'm' to phonology. An operational independence of the two routes is implied.

Case V.3 Mark T (born December 1966)

1 Psycho-educational background

Mark had a difficult birth (a face presentation) and suffered a mild encephalitis following measles innoculation at 1 year. Some brain damage was suspected and this diagnosis was supported by the results of an EEG investigation. At the time of referral to the Tayside Dyslexia Association in 1978 Mark was receiving drug therapy for the control of temper tantrums. An administration of the Similarities, Vocabulary, Block design and Object assembly sub-tests of the WISC gave scaled scores of 9, 11, 10 and 12, suggesting an average level of intelligence without a marked verbal-performance discrepancy. Reading and spelling assessments, carried out in 1978, 1979 and 1981, gave the results shown in Table 8.41. These indicate a retardation in both areas, especially spelling. The psychologist noted that Mark was left-handed and that he suffered an astygmatism in the left eye. He considered that his errors in reading and spelling were indicative of a mild dyslexic condition. A left-right confusion was also noted. The recommendation was that Mark should receive intensive remedial tuition in reading and spelling. At the start of the project in 1981 Mark was in his third year at secondary school. He was receiving remedial tuition in mathematics but not in English. He reported that the school was very sympathetic to his problems. His mother said that she also had spelling problems and tended to mix up the order of letters. Mark reads a lot and has an ambition to go into the navy after leaving school.

TABLE 8.41 *Results of administration of tests to subject MT (a) in 1978 when subject's CA was 11-6 years, and (b) in 1979 when subject's CA was 12-2 years, and (c) in 1981 when subject's CA was 14-8 years*

	Reading tests			Spelling tests	
a	Neale Analysis			Daniels and Diack	
	rate	9-3	years		8-1 years
	accuracy	9-4	years		
	comprehension	9-10	years		
b	Neale Analysis			Daniels and Diack	
	rate	9-3	years		8-3 years
	accuracy	9-4	years		
	comprehension	11-10	years		
c	Schonell			Schonell	
		12-10	years		8-1 years

2   Experimental data

Table 8.42 summarises MT's results for reading high frequency words, low frequency words and non-words. A large phonological effect is evident. The error rate for non-word reading approached 30 per cent and was significantly greater than the rates for high or low frequency words. Reaction time in non-word reading averaged over 4000 ms. The distribution, displayed in Figure 8.8, was widely dispersed (Type C distribution). The lexicality effect was over 2000 ms.

The results also give evidence of a morphemic dyslexia. The distributions for both high and low frequency words included a tail of slow responses (Type B distribution) and the error rates were somewhat above the range for competent readers. Nonetheless, the phonological effect seems substantially greater than the morphemic effect.

The analysis of the results for word reading showed no clear effects for the syntactic and semantic variables. Irregularity did not affect reaction

TABLE 8.42   *Vocal reaction times (ms) and error rates for reading high frequency words, low frequency words and non-words by MT*

| | High frequency words | | | Low frequency words | | | Non-words | | |
	Overall	Intercept	Slope	Overall	Intercept	Slope	Overall	Intercept	Slope
X̄	1437	1052	81	1801	838	209[1]	4018	298	785[1]
sd	770			1076			2721		
Error %	5.95			13.49			29.66		

[1] Linear trend significant at p<0.05 or better by F-test
Frequency effect t(265) = 3.207, p<0.005. $\chi^2(1)$ = 4.907, p<0.05
Lexicality effect (HF v NW):t(322) = 11.454, p<0.001. $\chi^2(1)$ 34.736, p<0.001
(LF v NW):t(273) = 8.069, p<0.001. $\chi^2(1)$ = 11.763, p<0.001

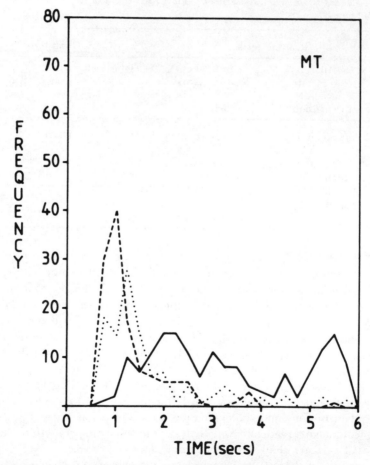

FIGURE 8.8   *Reaction time distributions for responses to high frequency words (– – –), low frequency words (. . .) and non-words (———) by MT*

time but did raise error rate from 3.57 per cent to 21.43 per cent for low frequency words (p<0.05). This suggests that, despite the phonological dyslexia, MT made use of route 'g' when attempting to read unfamiliar words. The occurrence of occasional regularisation errors (heir → 'hair', sew →'sue', corps → 'corpse', aisle → 'asel', heroism → 'hiroism', whereby →'wherebi') supports this conclusion. There were no derivational errors.

Non-word reading showed substantial effects of homophony which reduced the VRT from over 5000 ms to 3600 ms (p<0.01). This indicates that MT, like other phonologically dyslexic subjects, supported grapheme-phoneme translation by references to the lexicon. Nonetheless, more than half of his error responses were non-words.

TABLE 8.43 *Frequencies and latencies (ms) of word and non-word error responses to word and non-word targets by MT*

| | Words | | Non-words | |
	Words	Non-words	Words	Non-words
$\overline{\text{X}}$	1471	5004	3972	5718
sd	457	2175	1980	2611
N	14	13	27	43

Table 8.43 gives a breakdown of the frequencies of word and non-word error responses to word and non-word targets together with the error latencies. There was no significant tendency for error and target lexicality to covary or for one class of response to predominate over the other. There was a difference of over 4000 ms between word → word and non-word → non-word errors (p<0.001). This is consistent with the view that word → word errors (winter → 'winner', grief → 'chief', since → 'science') derive from confusions within the morphemic channel whereas non-word → non-word errors (poich → 'ponich', scrue → 'sucue', ose → 'ossy') are products of translation lapses within the slower grapheme-phoneme conversion channel. When the attempt to locate a word response to a word failed (e.g. freak →'frenk', lantern → 'lattern') the error latency rose to over 5000 ms. In these instances it is assumed that recognition by the input lexicon failed, attempts to locate a response in the output lexicon also failed, and that the eventual response was based on a phonology assembled within the translation channel. In the converse case, where a word response was made to a non-word target (e.g. spaich → 'spinach', thrish → 'thrush', drem → 'dream') the latency was 1700 ms shorter than for the non-word → non-word errors (p<0.01). This effect is presumed to have the same underlying mechanism as the homophony effect, that is to result from matching of output from the grapheme-phoneme channel against entries in the vocabulary store.

TABLE 8.44   *Reaction times (ms) and error rates for lexical and semantic decisions by MT*

			Lexical decisions			
		HF words	LF words	Legal non-words	Illegal non-words	All
	$\bar{X}$	1258	1694[2]	2488	1951	1739
	sd	734	909	1480	1164	1121
Error %		13.16	13.64	35	17.5	18.33
Rate (ms/letter)		263[1]		598	338	338[1]

[1] Significant linear trend
[2] Significant effect on reaction time
[3] Significant effect on error rate

It can be seen from the examples given that MT's error responses were generally structurally close to the target. The average similarity score was 66 per cent and over 80 per cent of errors had scores of 50 per cent or better. On the cluster by cluster analysis, accuracy was generally poorer on vowels than on consonants and on complex clusters than on simple clusters, falling from 75 per cent correct for simple consonants to 23 per cent correct for complex vowels. There was some evidence of use of correspondences above the grapheme-phoneme level. For example, halk was read as 'hawk'. About 15 per cent of responses showed evidence of the use of V+C correspondences. These data indicate that MT's translation channel was relatively accurate and sophisticated in its operation although the rate of handling information was extremely slow.

Table 8.44 gives a summary of the results of the lexical and semantic decision experiments. Semantic decisions were made somewhat slowly and the distribution was quite widely dispersed. Neither typicality nor relatedness exerted significant effects on reaction time or error rate. Lexical decisions were also made with reaction times and error rates somewhat above the normal range. The error rate of over 18 per cent included many incorrect responses to high frequency words and illegal non-words in addition to the more difficult low frequency words and legal non-words. One feature of MT's results is an absence of differentiation between legal and illegal non-words. These results suggest the presence of some inefficiency within route 'm' to semantics.

MT differed from SB and LT in that his phonological dyslexia was combined with a visual processor impairment. This was most strikingly evident in the visual matching tasks. The data, summarised in Table 8.45, show delays of response in both the identity matching and the array matching tasks. Mean reaction times were elevated in the format distortion and mirror letter versions of the identity matching task, and the processing rate for vertical displays was 92 ms/letter. Reaction times for array

Typical positives	Atypical positives	Semantic decisions Related negatives	Unrelated negatives	All
1820	1800	2640	2544	2215
777	622	1185	1933	1338
10.71	24.14	23.33	6.67	16.24
				132

matching, falling between 2800 ms and 4800 ms, were extremely slow and were combined with high error rates and dispersed distributions. There was no clear evidence of serial left-to-right processing. However, there was a large effect of legality (over 1500 ms) on positive reaction times.

TABLE 8.45 *Reaction times (ms) and error rates for visual matching tasks by MT*

Experiment		Identity matching Overall	Rate (ms/letter)		Array matching Overall	Position of difference (ms/position)
1	$\bar{X}$	1160	−5	$\bar{X}$	2801	159
	sd	676		sd	1683	
	Error %	6.67		Error %	26	
2	$\bar{X}$	1822	25	$\bar{X}$	4830	15
	sd	961		sd	2871	
	Error %	8.02		Error %	16.81	
3	$\bar{X}$	1853	18	$\bar{X}$	3405	268
	sd	1005		sd	1988	
	Error %	5		Error %	19.38	

[1] Linear trend significant at $p < 0.05$ or better by F-test

An absence of serial processing was also suggested by the analysis of word length effects. The rate for vocalisation of high frequency words was 80 ms/letter, but this reduced to 49 ms/letter when outlying responses were removed. In neither case was the test for linear trend significant. The rate for semantic decisions was also within the normal range. Unusually, positive lexical decisions were associated with a significant length effect of 263 ms/letter. The rate for non-word reading was very slow (over 700 ms/letter).

In certain respects, therefore, MT shows the same pattern of slow matching and absence of serial processing in word reading as occurred in the cases of visual analytic dyslexia described in Chapter 6. However, his results from the format distortion experiments, which appear in Table 8.46, were extremely variable and do not show the switch from parallel to slow serial processing which appeared in the data of RO and MF. There were no clear effects in the semantic decision task. Lexical decisions and vocal responses to low frequency words involved very slow serial processing for normal displays as well as for distorted displays. In the case of non-word reading, distortion appeared to interact with translation difficulty to produce processing rates in excess of 1000 ms/letter

TABLE 8.46   *Reaction times (ms) and error rates for reading normal and distorted words or non-words by MT*

		Vocalisation tasks		Decision tasks	
		Words	Non-words	Semantic	Lexical
Normal	X̄	2276	3625	1638	2524
	sd	1513	1731	749	1371
Error %		10	26.67	4.35	13.33
	Rate	469[1]	346	12	325[1]
Zigzag	X̄	3156	5721	2409[2]	3959[2]
	sd	2255	4253	1183	2121
Error %		6.67	33.33	12.77	20
	Rate	684[1]	1498[1]	69	448[1]
Vertical	X̄	2858	5176	2320[2]	3629[2]
	sd	1425	4163	1282	1966
Error %		23.33[1]	40	2.08	20
	Rate	377	1691[1]	113	488[1]

[1] Significant linear trend
[2] Format effect on reaction time
[3] Format effect on accuracy

3   Conclusions

MT's Level I description suggests that he is a boy of average ability who has encountered dyslexic difficulties in learning to read and spell which may be associated with neurological damage incurred early in life.

The Level II description indicates the presence of a severe phonological dyslexia combined with a visual processor dyslexia and somewhat milder effects on the morphemic routes to phonology and semantics. The details of this multiple impairment have been summarised in Table 8.47.

The impairment of route 'g' is similar to that shown by SB and LT. There was a very large effect on translation time. Nonetheless, a procedure for grapheme-phoneme conversion existed and was used in non-word

TABLE 8.47   *Summary of cognitive description of reading functions of subject MT*

'm' → phonology	Impaired	Large frequency effect. Grapheme-phoneme support for low frequency words. Regularisation errors
'g' → phonology	Very impaired	Lexical support. Difficulty with complex vowels. Occasional use of V+C correspondences
'm' → semantics	Impaired	Absence of legality effect. Serial processing in lexical decisions
Visual processor	Impaired	Slow identity matching. Slow array matching. Orthographic model. Disruption by format distortion

reading and as occasional support for word retrieval. Inaccuracies of translation were generally minor failures of correspondence which focused in particular on complex graphemic structures. Co-operation between the 'm' and 'g' routes to phonology was suggested by the occurrence of regularity effects and regularisation errors in word reading and by the effect of homophony on non-word reading.

MT's visual processor impairment appeared fairly diffuse. There was no general disturbance of the wholistic function. However, the analytic tasks of matching and format distortion resolution showed large effects.

Case V.4   Joanna B (born March 1969)

1   Psycho-educational background

Joanna was born at home at full term after a long labour. She was slow to breathe on account of a complication (cord around her neck). Subsequent developmental milestones were somewhat delayed. She walked at 24 months and produced single words at 2-6 years. Her early childhood was healthy apart from occasional earache. The family, which included an older brother and sister, moved from the south of England to Scotland when Joanna was 4 years old. Her parents suspected learning difficulties when she entered primary school at the age of 5 years. She received remedial help at school and also attended for speech therapy up to the age of 8 years. Her school reports commented on a lack of confidence. JB is left-handed, although her parents were not aware of this until she started at school. Her father commented that he had experienced difficulty in learning to read. He campaigned to persuade JB's secondary school to allow concessions in examinations. It was agreed that the questions should be recorded and played to Joanna so that she should not have to read them. At the present time she is preparing to sit four subjects at the 'O' Grade (Cooking, Art,

Arithmetic and English). Her hobbies are reading (mainly romances and thrillers), sewing, lace making, swimming, ski-ing and helping with the Brownies. She is able to type and hopes to find a position using this skill.

JB's parents approached the Tayside Dyslexia Association in 1981 on the advice of a health visitor. An intellectual assessment was made using an abbreviated WISC. Performance IQ was assessed as average and verbal IQ as somewhat below average. The lowest score was on the digit span sub-test. A reassessment in 1984 confirmed the results of the earlier testing. The sub-test scores appear in Table 8.48.

TABLE 8.48   *Results of the administration of the WISC to subject JB (a) in 1981 when subject's CA was 11-11 years, and (b) in 1984 when subject's CA was 15-7 years*

	Verbal tests		Performance tests	
	Similarities	8	Block design	9
a	Vocabulary	10	Object assembly	12
	Digit span	7		
	Verbal IQ	94	Performance IQ	102
	Information	5	Picture completion	8
	Similarities	7	Picture arrangement	13
b	Arithmetic	5	Block design	9
	Vocabulary	8	Object assembly	11
	Comprehension	13	Coding	12
	Digit span	8		
	Verbal IQ	85	Performance IQ	104

TABLE 8.49   *Results of administration of reading and spelling tests to subject JB (a) in 1981 when subject's CA was 11-11 years, and (b) in 1984 when subject's CA was 15-7 years*

	Reading tests		Spelling tests	
	Neale Analysis		Daniels and Diack (test 11)	
	rate	8-5 years		8-7 years
	accuracy	8-6 years		
a	comprehension	9-1 years		
	Daniels and Diack (test 12)			
		9-5 years		
	Schonell (test A)		Schonell	
		10-5 years		9-8 years
b	Daniels and Diack (test 12)			
		12-1 years		
	Schonell (R4 test)			
		14 years		

JB's reading was assessed in 1981 and 1984. The results, summarised in Table 8.49, show that she was between 2 and 3 years behind her chronological age at the first testing. The subsequent testing indicated progress in the area of reading comprehension although basic word recognition skills, as assessed by the Schonell test, remained impaired. She made visual and derivational errors on the tests and scored poorly on a test of nonsense word reading (13/22). The table also gives the results of formal tests of spelling. It is clear that her spelling remained seriously impaired throughout the period of the investigation. The educational psychologist commented that the errors showed poor auditory discrimination and incorrect sound-symbol association. JB's writing was reported to be neat, with satisfactory volume of output, punctuation and content. She writes left-handed, holding the page at 90 degrees. Occasional b-d reversals were noted.

Visual functions were tested by administration of the Graham Kendall Memory for Designs test in 1981 and 1984. No impairment was noted on either occasion. In 1984 she attended an opthalmic clinic for tests of visual functions. Her vision was reported to be normal although an application of the Dunlop test suggested that she had not established a stable reference eye.

Auditory functions were tested in 1981 using the Wepman test. Her score was below the threshold of adequacy at the 8-year level and revealed problems of discrimination affecting the high frequency sounds (/v/, /f/, /θ/, /ʃ/). However, subsequent testing using pure tone and speech audiometry procedures revealed no impairment. The Lindamood Auditory Conceptualisation test was administered in 1984. Joanna scored 70/100. This is a level appropriate for a Primary 3 child and was taken by the educational psychologist to indicate a severe problem in operating on the component sounds of words.

The items from the Bangor Dyslexia test were administered in 1984. There were positive indications on 8/10 items, including left-right discrimination, repetition of polysyllables, recall of multiplication tables, the months sequence and digit span. The psychologist also noted some word-finding difficulties and confusions over word structure (e.g. 'workclock' for clockwork) and tenses ('he's had to fought for me').

2 Experimental data

Table 8.50 summarises JB's results for reading high frequency words, low frequency words and non-words. The distributions of correct reaction times appear in Figure 8.9. The data are indicative of a severe combined phonological and morphemic dyslexia. The 'phonological dyslexia' is indicated by the high error rate in non-word reading (over 40 per cent) and by the extreme elevation of the reaction time and dispersal of the distribution. The lexicality effect was over 1600 ms. The 'morphemic dyslexia' is suggested by (1) the high error rate and tail of slow responses (Type B distribution) for high frequency word reading, and (2) the very high error rate (over 36 per cent) for low frequency words and the extreme dispersion of the reaction times (Type C distribution). There was a large difference between high and low frequency words (over 2000 ms).

The analysis of psycholinguistic effects yielded a standard configuration for phonological dyslexia. JB did not show any consistent effects of spelling-to-sound regularity but there were some effects of abstract versus concrete meaning. These have been summarised in Table 8.51. Unlike LT, JB did not show effects of form class. However, abstract meaning was associated with a significant rise in error rate and with very slow responses to lower frequency words. This suggests that semantic processing was sometimes involved in word retrieval but that there was no consistent reliance on the defective grapheme-phoneme translation channel.

TABLE 8.50   *Vocal reaction times (ms) and error rates for reading high frequency words, low frequency words and non-words by JB*

| | High frequency words | | | Low frequency words | | | Non-words | | |
	Overall	Intercept	Slope	Overall	Intercept	Slope	Overall	Intercept	Slope
X̄	1612	868	161[1]	3685	1279	521	5298	2636	548[1]
sd	874			3706			3027		
Error %	14.88			36.51			41.95		

[1] Linear trend significant at p<0.05 or better by F-test
Frequency effect: t(221) = 6.349, p<0.001. $\chi^2(1)$ = 18.385, p<0.001
Lexicality effect (HF v NW):t(278) = 13.913, p<0.001. $\chi^2(1)$ = 33.802, p<0.001
(LF v NW):t(215) =   3.464, p<0.001. $\chi^2(1)$ = 1.013

TABLE 8.51   *Reaction times (ms) and error rates for reading function words and concrete and abstract words of high and low frequency by JB*

| | High frequency words | | | Low frequency words | |
	Function	Concrete	Abstract	Concrete	Abstract
X̄	1644	1511	1834	3266	8630[1]
sd	762	733	927	1494	7663
Error %	11.9	4.76	28.57[2]	28.57	57.14

[1] Significant effect on reaction time
[2] Significant effect on accuracy

JB's non-word reading was affected by homophony which reduced error rate from 48 to 30 per cent (p<0.05) and reaction time from 6900 ms to 4200 ms (p<0.001). This implies that output from the translation channel was sometimes 'lexicalised' by reference to the speech production vocabulary store. However, JB, like the other subjects, both read a

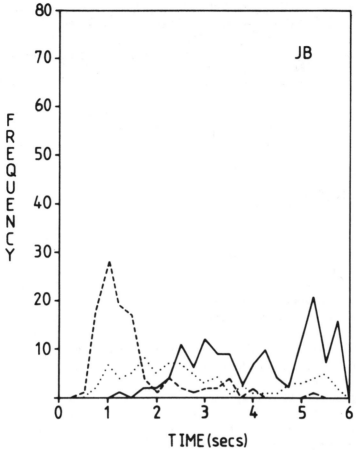

FIGURE 8.9   *Reaction time distributions for responses to high frequency words (– – –), low frequency words (. . .) and non-words (——) by JB*

substantial number of non-words correctly and produced non-word error responses. This is documented in Table 8.52 which gives the frequencies and latencies of word and non-word error responses to word and non-word targets. Overall, JB showed a bias in favour of production of word responses (p<0.001). However, this was attributable mainly to responses to words. Reponses to non-words were more evenly divided. The error reaction times were all very high (in excess of 5000 ms). This suggests that a majority of errors probably involved attempts to read via the translation channel. Like the other subjects, JB produced responses which were in approximate correspondence with their targets (average similarity score = 61 per cent). Mis-translations focused on the complex graphemic structures, particularly the vowels. JB's error set included only one phonetic regularisation (isle → 'izzle') but several derivational errors (heroism → 'hero',   loyalty → 'loyal',   greed → 'greedy',   these → 'those', variety → 'vary', drunk → 'drink', and won → 'win').

TABLE 8.52   *Frequencies and latencies (ms) of word and non-word error responses to word and non-word targets by JB*

	Words		Non-words	
	Words	Non-words	Words	Non-words
X̄	5559	13333	6526	7114
sd	4769	10780	3214	3804
N	56	15	55	44

[1] Significant linear trend
[2] Significant effect on reaction time

JB's performance on the lexical and semantic decisions tasks has been summarised in Tables 8.53 and 8.54. Lexical decisions were made with a reaction time slightly above the competent reader range and a high rate of error (65 per cent) on the legal non-words. The legality effects on negative RT were significant but there was no effect of frequency. Semantic decision RT and error rate were also slightly elevated relative to the results of the competent readers. There were clear effects of both typicality and relatedness on reaction time and error rates. These results are somewhat equivocal regarding the status of route 'm' to semantics, but suggest that the route was either efficient or only quite mildly impaired.

TABLE 8.53   *Reaction times (ms) and error data for lexical decisions by JB*

	HF words	LF words	Legal non-words	Illegal non-words	All
X̄	1345	1533	2211[2]	1527	1511
sd	618	387	916	323	555
Error %	5.26	18.18	65[3]	2.5	16.67
Rate		24	−86	39	4

[1] Significant linear trend
[2] Significant effect on reaction time
[3] Significant effect on error rate.

The analysis of visual processor functions was also suggestive of a general absence of impairment. Table 8.55 gives the results from the visual matching tasks. Both identity matching and array matching were carried out with reaction times and error rates which fell within or close to the normal range. There were no clear effects of orthographic legality on reaction time in the array matching task.

TABLE 8.54 *Reaction times (ms) and error rates for semantic decisions by JB*

	Typical positives	Atypical positives	Related negatives	Unrelated negatives	All
$\bar{X}$	1479	1846^2	2116^2	1735	1769
sd	459	654	621	391	572
Error %	3.45	36.67^3	26.67^3	0	16.95
Rate (ms/letter)					28

[1] Significant linear trend
[2] Significant effect on reaction time
[3] Significant effect on error rate

TABLE 8.55 *Reaction times (ms) and error rates for visual matching tasks by JB*

Experiment		Identity matching			Array matching	
		Overall	Rate (ms/letter)		Overall	Position of difference (ms/position)
1	$\bar{X}$	918	12	$\bar{X}$	1255	49
	sd	263		sd	378	
	Error %	0.83		Error %	7	
2	$\bar{X}$	934	19^1	$\bar{X}$	1490	183^1
	sd	280		sd	578	
	Error %	1.85		Error %	10	
3	$\bar{X}$	873	-3	$\bar{X}$	1915	108^1
	sd	314		sd	680	
	Error %	2.5		Error %	3.13	

[1] Linear trend significant at $p < 0.05$ or better by F-test

There was also no strong evidence of serial processing in JB's reading. No consistent length effects occurred in the lexical and semantic decisions tasks. Vocalisation of high frequency words involved a relatively slow rate of 160 ms/letter. However, an analysis based on reaction times below 2000 ms, which form the main body of JB's distribution for high frequency words, gave a rate of 70 ms/letter. As is typical in phonological dyslexia, the rate for non-words was considerably slower (over 500 ms/letter).

Table 8.56 gives the results for the format distortion experiments. The data from the decision tasks suggest that JB was generally able to resolve the distortions without a switch to slow serial processing. The results from the vocalisation tasks were more variable. Extremely slow processing rates occurred for non-word reading. The slope values for words were substantial but generally did not reflect consistent linear trends. It seems probable that these effects were connected with JB's phonological impairment. No general

TABLE 8.56   *Reaction times (ms) and error rates for reading normal and distorted words or non-words by JB*

		Vocalisation tasks		Decision tasks	
		Words	Non-words	Semantic	Lexical
Normal	$\bar{X}$	1850	6040	1346	1502
	sd	1045	3436	679	583
Error %		26.67	36.67	12.5	20
	Rate	210	1243[1]	89	32
Zigzag	$\bar{X}$	2779[2]	4993	1626	1672
	sd	1519	2609	941	618
Error %		20	46.67	12.5	23.33
	Rate	262	1060[1]	231[1]	17
Vertical	$\bar{X}$	3941[2]	6400	1590	1656
	sd	2583	3109	700	508
Error %		30	43.33	16.67	26.67
	Rate	641	1253[1]	86	51

[1] Significant linear trend
[2] Format effect on reaction time
[3] Format effect on accuracy

impairment of the capability of the visual processor to resolve distortions is indicated.

3   Conclusions

JB's Level I description suggests that she is a girl of average non-verbal ability and slightly below average verbal ability who has suffered quite severe dyslexic difficulties in acquiring reading and spelling skills. Accompanying defects in auditory conceptualisation are indicated.

Her Level II description is indicative of a phonological dyslexia as the predominant feature together with a relatively severe morphemic effect. A summary of the conclusions appears in Table 8.57. The overall configuration is similar to that proposed for SB and LT in that effects on the 'g' and 'm' routes to phonology are combined with a relative sparing of the visual processor and route 'm' to semantics.

JB exhibits a number of characteristics which also appeared in the data of LT. Her reading of words was not affected by regularity but did show some semantic effects. Derivational paralexias occurred in her error set. These results are consistent with the proposal that word reading was supported by some semantic processes. Like LT, JB possessed an operational grapheme-phoneme translator which she used when attempting to read non-words. The translator functioned extremely slowly and somewhat inaccurately with support from the speech production lexicon.

The observation that route 'm' to semantics was relatively unimpaired whereas there was a severe effect on route 'm' to phonology supports the

TABLE 8.57   *Summary of cognitive description of reading functions of subject JB*

Function	Status	Comment
'm' → phonology	Very impaired	Very large frequency effect. Semantic processing support. Bias in favour of word errors. Derivational errors. Fast serial processing
'g' → phonology	Very impaired	Lexical support. Slow serial processing
'm' → semantics	Mildly impaired?	Inaccurate on legal non-words. Effects of typicality and relatedness. Slow
Visual processor	Efficient	Slow format resolution for non-words

proposal in favour of the differentiation between the two morphemic routes. The results also favour the view that the manner in which the visual processor functions may be dictated by the higher level process which is being accessed. When route 'm' to semantics was involved processing appeared parallel and the distortions were tolerated without notable costs. Phonological access, especially via route 'g', results in serial processing and an exaggeration of the distortion effects.

Case V.5   Paul S (born June 1969)

1   Psycho-educational background

Paul S was born six weeks prematurely by Caesarian section. Motor and linguistic development during the pre-school period were reported as normal. He is right-handed but this was a matter of some uncertainty during his primary schooling. Clock time was not mastered until the age of 12 years. His parents were aware of learning difficulties from Primary 1 onwards and his school reports noted problems with reading and number despite good effort. He was regarded as a 'slow learner' by his teachers. An assessment was made by the Tayside Dyslexia Association in 1981 and following this he received individual tuition for about two years. His secondary school arranged for him to have supplementary lessons in spelling. His reports consistently praise his effort and attitude to work. He enjoys athletics, woodwork and computer games but does not read for pleasure. His parents and two siblings were also reported to have experienced learning difficulties.

Paul's general intelligence was assessed in 1981 using an abbreviated version of the WISC. An average level of ability was suggested (Full scale IQ = 96) with no marked verbal-performance discrepancy. Administration of the full set of sub-tests in 1984 confirmed the earlier results. The scores appear in Table 8.58. The psychologist commented on the marked weakness on the digit span test of auditory sequential memory and on the superior performance on the object assembly test. This was regarded as consistent with Paul's statement that he enjoyed working with his hands and that he would like to find a career using these skills.

TABLE 8.58   *Results of administrations of the WISC to subject PS (a) in 1981 when subject's CA was 11-8 years, and (b) in 1984 when subject's CA was 15-4 years*

	Verbal tests		Performance tests	
	Similarities	9	Block design	11
a	Vocabulary	10	Object assembly	10
	Digit span	8		
	Verbal IQ	**94**	**Performance IQ**	**103**
	Information	10	Picture completion	12
b	Similarities	11	Picture arrangement	11
	Arithmetic	10	Block design	10
	Vocabulary	12	Object assembly	15
	Comprehension	9	Coding	9
	Digit span	6		
	Verbal IQ	**102**	**Performance IQ**	**109**

TABLE 8.59   *Results of administration of reading and spelling tests to subject PS (a) in 1981 when subject's CA was 11-8 years, and (b) in 1984 when subject's CA was 15-4 years*

	Reading tests		Spelling tests	
	Neale Analysis		Daniels and Diack	
a	rate	9-0 years		7-8 years
	accuracy	9-0 years		
	comprehension	10-11 years		
	Schonell (test A)		Schonell (test A)	
		12-0 years		11-1 years
b	Daniels and Diack (test 12)			
		14+ years		
	Schonell (R4B test)			
		11-2 years		

PS's reading was assessed in 1981 by means of the Neale Analysis of Reading. His age scores, reported in Table 8.59, show a retardation of over 2 years on the rate and accuracy measures. The scores on the tests applied in 1984 reveal a definite progress in the intervening period. Comprehension under untimed conditions was at ceiling. The lower score on the timed test was taken to be a consequence of his slowness in reading. In the single word test he made visual, derivational and occasional semantically influenced errors (choir → 'chorus'). He scored only 11/22 on a test of reading nonsense words, suggesting a severe weakness in phonological assembly.

Table 8.59 also gives results of spelling assessments. In 1981 his spelling age was 7-8 years and had risen to over 11 years in 1984. Errors included refusals and partial responses, confusion over double letters and omissions. His free writing was limited in quantity of output and involved poor spelling and sentence structure, inappropriate use of capitals, absence of punctuation and occasional b-d confusions and malformation of letters.

In 1981 the educational psychologist commented that PS used 'short sentences with almost telegrammatic phrases' and recommended that the opinion of the school speech therapist be sought. After an interview the speech therapist reported that Paul was relaxed and 'chatty' and that no articulative defects were present. He was tested on the Illinois Test of Psycholinguistic Abilities (ITPA) and showed a composite psycholinguistic age of 9-7 years. The speech therapist commented that his score on the Verbal Expression test was particularly poor although she did not consider that speech therapy would be beneficial. In 1984 PS was assessed by the Lindamood Auditory Conceptualisation test. His score of 88/100 was considered predictive of reading and spelling difficulties in a child at the upper primary level and as suggestive of a weakness in the ability to operate on the component sounds of words.

In responding to the items from the Bangor test, PS had difficulty with the months sequence, the tables and the repetition of polysyllables. His score of 7 on the test was considered positive, i.e. an indication that he exhibited the pattern of extrinsic signs often associated with dyslexia. Tests of visual functions did not give evidence of impairments. His score on the Graham Kendall Memory for Designs test was normal. Orthoptics testing indicated that he had established his right eye as a dominant reference eye and that his vision was normal.

Experimental data

Table 8.60 gives a summary of PS's results for reading high frequency words, low frequency words and non-words. A plot of the reaction time distributions appears in Figure 8.10.

The results give a clear indication of a 'phonological dyslexia'. The error rate in non-word reading approached 30 per cent. Reaction times for non-words were extremely slow and dispersed, with a preponderance of times in excess of 5000 ms. The lexicality effect was over 2500 ms.

PS's data are also indicative of a 'morphemic dyslexia'. The error rates for reading both high and low frequency words were elevated at 11 and 18 per cent. The reaction time for reading high frequency words was very

TABLE 8.60   *Vocal reaction times (ms) and error rates for reading high frequency words, low frequency words and non-words by PS*

| | High frequency words | | | Low frequency words | | | Non-words | | |
	Overall	Intercept	Slope	Overall	Intercept	Slope	Overall	Intercept	Slope
X̄	2209	1248	206	3291	1828	316	5856	1364	951[1]
sd	2098			2574			4043		
Error %	11.31			18.25			29.66		

[1] Linear trend significant at p<0.05 or better by F-test

Frequency effect: $t(250) = 3.648$, p<0.001. $\chi^2(1) = 2.836$

Lexicality effect (HF v NW): $t(313) = 9.848$, p<0.001. $\chi^2(1) = 19.848$, p<0.001

(LF v NW): $t(267) = 5.733$, p<0.001. $\chi^2(1) = 5.599$, p<0.02

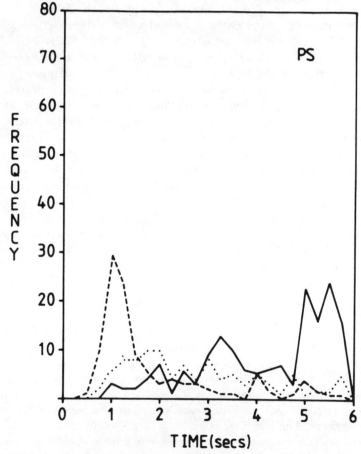

FIGURE 8.10   *Reaction time distributions for responses to high frequency words (– – –), low frequency words (. . .) and non-words (——) by PS*

high at over 2200 ms and formed a Type B distribution containing a substantial tail of slow responses. There was a frequency effect of over 1000 ms. Low frequency words had a latency of over 3200 ms and the reaction times were widely dispersed with no preponderance of fast times (Type C distribution).

The analysis of the effects of the psycholinguistic factors was inconclusive. Neither form class nor abstract meaning nor spelling-to-sound irregularity produced reliable effects on reaction time or accuracy. Hence, the data do not give clear indications of support by semantic processing or grapheme-phoneme translation during word retrieval. PS's error set included only two possible regularisations but five clear derivational paralexias (society → 'socially', anger → 'angry', life → 'live', hunger → 'hungry', muscle → 'muscular').

Non-word homophony did not influence the accuracy or the latency of responses to non-words. This suggests that PS did not attempt to 'lexicalise' output from his impaired grapheme-phoneme translation channel. The availability of the channel is suggested by the occurrence of non-word error responses to both word and non-word targets. About 50 per cent of incorrect responses to words were non-words, and over 67 per cent of responses to non-words. Error responses were made with a very high latency (over 7800 ms), suggesting that many of them were produced after attempts to use the impaired translation channel. The structural analysis of errors supported the general finding that mis-translations focus on the complex graphemic clusters, especially the vowels. Only 21 per cent of complex vowels were correctly translated, as against 57 per cent of complex consonants.

Table 8.61 gives a summary of the results from the lexical and semantic decision tasks. Semantic decisions were made quite accurately (8 per cent error rate) but the reaction time was elevated. The distribution has been plotted in Figure 8.11 and can be seen to be extremely widely dispersed. There were no consistent effects of typicality or relatedness. A similar picture was presented by the lexical decision data. Performance was reasonably accurate but the mean reaction time exceeded 3200 ms and the distribution was widely dispersed. There was an effect of legality on the negative RT, but responses to the illegal non-words were extremely slow (over 3400 ms). These results provide clear indications of an impairment of route 'm' to semantics.

The analysis of PS's visual processor suggested the presence of an impairment of the wholistic function. There were large effects of word length on responses to words in the lexical decision task (over 500 ms/letter) and in the semantic decision task (330 ms/letter). Following removal of outliers >4000 ms the rate for vocalisation of high frequency words was found to be 142 ms/letter. There was an extremely large effect on non-word reading (over 950 ms/letter).

TABLE 8.61 *Reaction times (ms) and error data for lexical and semantic decisions by PS*

| | | | Lexical decisions | | |
	HF words	LF words	Legal non-words	Illegal non-words	All
$\bar{X}$	1867	2661	6728[2]	3462	3218
sd	1604	2587	2312	2456	2691
Error %	0	13.64[3]	25	5	8.33
Rate (ms/letter)	537[1]		107	−352	92

[1] Significant linear trend
[2] Significant effect on reaction time
[3] Significant effect on error rate

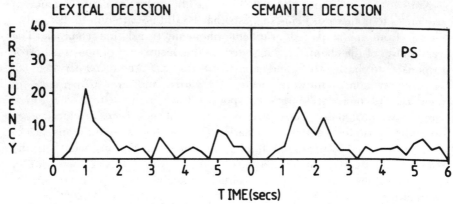

FIGURE 8.11 *Reaction time distributions for lexical and semantic decisions by PS*

TABLE 8.62 *Reaction times (ms) and error rates for visual matching tasks by PS*

| Experiment | | Identity matching | | | Array matching | |
		Overall	Rate (ms/letter)		Overall	Position of difference (ms/position)
1	$\bar{X}$	1038	21[1]	$\bar{X}$	2148	95
	sd	260		sd	481	
	Error %	0		Error %	4	
2	$\bar{X}$	1108	6	$\bar{X}$	2487	174[1]
	sd	315		sd	778	
	Error %	0		Error %	3.33	
3	$\bar{X}$	1151	−14	$\bar{X}$	2881	110[1]
	sd	306		sd	643	
	Error %	0		Error %	1.25	

[1] Linear trend significant at $p < 0.05$ or better by F-test

Typical positives	Atypical positives	Semantic decisions Related negatives	Unrelated negatives	All
1953	2702	4301	3928	3246
1056	2104	2472	2884	2439
3.45	17.24	6.67	3.33	7.63
				332[1]

The results from the visual matching tasks have been summarised in Table 8.62. Identity matching performance was efficient, with no errors and reaction times lying at the upper end of the normal range. Array matching, although accurate, involved reaction times somewhat above the normal range (2100-2800 ms). This suggests the possibility of an impairment to the analytic function of the visual processor. There was a legality effect of over 360 ms on positive RT (p<0.01).

TABLE 8.63 *Reaction times (ms) and error rates for reading normal and distorted words or non-words by PS*

		Vocalisation tasks Words	Non-words	Decision tasks Semantic	Lexical
Normal	$\bar{X}$	2168	4767	2526	2740
	sd	1560	1732	2387	2362
Error %		20	30	2.08	16.67
	Rate	263	98	517[1]	370
Zigzag	$\bar{X}$	4081[2]	8206[2]	2926	4181[2]
	sd	3216	6217	3163	3309
Error %		6.67	30	10.87	21.67
	Rate	1264[1]	2314[1]	902[1]	685[1]
Vertical	$\bar{X}$	4267[2]	11623[2]	3079	5058[2]
	sd	4144	7980	1885	5284
Error %		26.67	26.67	4.26	13.33
	Rate	1304[1]	3008[1]	425[1]	1394[1]

[1] Significant linear trend
[2] Format effect on reaction time
[3] Format effect on accuracy

Table 8.63 gives the results for the format distortion experiments. These data were extremely variable but suggest the involvement of very slow serial processing which was vulnerable to distortion. The effect was most strikingly evident in the non-word reading task where processing rates rose 2-3 seconds per letter. The general impression is that the need to resolve the distortions caused an extreme disruption of PS's visual processor functions.

3   Conclusions

PS's Level I description identifies him as a boy of average general ability who has suffered severe difficulties in establishing basic reading and spelling skills. There is an indication of accompanying disabilities affecting auditory conceptualisation and short-term sequential memory.

The Level II description, which has been summarised in Table 8.64, shows the presence of a severe multiple impairment affecting all four processing domains. PS has a major phonological dyslexia which is marked by slow, serial and inaccurate translation of non-words via route 'g' to phonology. He also shows large morphemic impairments which are indexed by (1) slowness of semantic access in the categorisation and lexical decision experiments (effect on route 'm' to semantics), and (2) slow and inaccurate vocalisation of words of lower frequency (effect on route 'm' to phonology). There are in addition indications of impairments to the visual processor affecting its capacity to operate in wholistic mode and its speed of handling information in analytic mode.

TABLE 8.64   *Summary of cognitive description of reading functions of subject PS*

Function	Status	Comment
'm' → phonology	Very impaired	Derivational errors. Slow serial processing
'g' → phonology	Very impaired	Difficulty with complex vowels. Very slow serial processing
'm' → semantics	Impaired reaction time	Slow responses to illegal non-words. Very slow serial processing
Visual processor	Impaired	Slow array matching. Orthographic model. Large distortion effects

Conclusions: Series V

The Series V subjects all presented with severe difficulties in non-word reading which were taken to be indicative of a major impairment of route 'g' to phonology. They are, in this sense, cases of 'phonological dyslexia', although it is evident from the detailed analyses that quite considerable heterogeneity existed at the level of comparisons between processing configurations.

Two of the subjects, MT and PS, provide demonstrations of multiply impaired systems in which inefficiencies occurred in all four domains. The other three, SB, LT and JB, gave evidence of more narrowly localised impairments affecting the 'g' and 'm' routes to phonology but not route 'm' to semantics or the visual processor.

8.4   Conclusions

The subjects whose cases were discussed in this chapter showed large effects on non-word reading. According to the assumptions of the research, they all gave evidence of an impairment of route 'g' to phonology. By examining the similarities and differences between their Level II descriptions it is possible to determine whether 'phonological dyslexia' can be identified with a particular processing configuration.

There were some common features which were represented in the data of all the subjects. In each case route 'g' was impaired in speed of functioning but was nonetheless an operational system which was used in some reading tasks. There was also an accompanying impairment of route 'm' to phonology. The configuration under discussion therefore consisted of a combined effect on the 'm' and 'g' routes to phonology, with the impact on route 'g' being the more severe.

The results indicate that the presence of this dual impairment did not have consistent implications for the states of the remaining two elements of the cognitive analysis, the visual processor and route 'm' to semantics. Subjects SM, LT and JB presented a configuration in which these two elements functioned quite efficiently. The remaining subjects, JM, SE, MP, MT and PS, showed impairments in these systems as well as in the routes of phonology.

The question of the relationship between the 'g' and 'm' routes to phonology is difficult to resolve. It could be that there is some common adverse factor located in the phonological processor which impaired both processes, although to differing degrees. Alternatively, it is possible that a severe effect on route 'g' has damaging implications for route 'm'. Finally, it could be that two quite independent effects of variable impact are involved. The principal counter-argument to the first two possibilities is the observation that Series I subjects, such as AD and SS, showed effects on route 'g' in the absence of effects on route 'm'. This issue will be taken up again in the next chapter.

Another question is whether a phonological dyslexia has a consistent influence on the compensatory reading strategies adopted by a subject. As was noted at the beginning of this chapter, a standard view is that route 'g' should not be used to support word retrieval and that there should be a consequent reliance on lexical and semantic processing. This account predicts that phonological dyslexia should be characterised by (1) an absence of spelling-to-sound regularity effects and phonetic regularisation errors, (2) an influence of semantic and syntactic variables on word retrieval, and (3) a predominance of words among error responses and the occurrence of some derivational or semantic errors.

The data suggest that this account, which derives from the analysis of acquired phonological dyslexia, is not applicable to developmental cases of the type considered here. The two best approximations are subjects LT and JB who combined the absence of regularity effects with semantic effects on reading and the production of some derivational errors. Most of the other subjects were sensitive to the regularity variable. This implies that they made some use of the translation channel in reading, although, in the cases of JM and SB, there was also evidence of semantic back-up processing.

All subjects other than PS were influenced by non-word homophony. Thus it appears that the most commonly adopted strategy was one of supporting grapheme-phoneme translation by access to stored vocabulary. In subjects JM, SE, MP, SB and MT the homophony effect was combined with a regularity effect, suggesting that the 'g' and 'm' routes operated on a basis of mutual support. It seems likely that in this subject sample the impairment of route 'g' was simply not severe enough to force a resort to fully lexicalised or semantic reading. Even the most severely affected subjects, JB and PS, possessed operational grapheme-phoneme translators which produced an acceptable output on a substantial proportion of non-words (60-70 per cent). Error responses were, for the most part, reasonable approximations to the targets and many of them were non-words.

9 Conclusions and prospects

9.1 Introduction

In the introductory chapters to this monograph I argued that 'dyslexia', defined as a disability affecting the acquisition of basic reading and spelling skills, would benefit from an analysis based on the application of a cognitive experimental method. This method involved (1) the formulation of a functional model of basic reading processes, (2) the construction of a set of tasks and factor variations which were calculated to provide information about the component processes specified in the model, and (3) the application of the experimental procedure to the individual members of a subject sample.

A simple model, based on the notion of interaction between visual, semantic and phonological processors, was outlined in Chapter 2. Chapters 3 and 4 described an associated experimental procedure designed to obtain reaction time and accuracy data in the context of vocalisation and decision tasks which incorporated appropriate factor variations.

The remainder of the monograph has described the results of an application of the procedure to (1) a sample of competent 11-year-old readers, and (2) a series of dyslexic cases aged 12 years and above. The results of the competent readers provided a basis for estimates of the characteristics of efficient performance on each of the experimental tasks. The main objective was to formulate a 'cognitive description' of the processing system established by each of the dyslexic subjects. These descriptions were viewed as interpretations of the experimental data, formulated by reference to the model, which specified the status (efficient or impaired) of each component and gave information about functional characteristics.

9.2   Levels of description

The accounts of the cases were formulated at two levels, referred to as Level I and Level II descriptions. The Level I descriptions were statements of the competence of each individual in reading and spelling and wider areas of ability as determined by informed observation and the application of standardised test instruments. Such descriptions are essential for the public definition of 'dyslexia' and constitute a necessary preliminary step in diagnosis. However, they do not provide an adequate basis for a functional (information processing) account of impaired reading processes. It would be unwise to assume that sub-test patterns on the WISC or other scales could confidently be taken to indicate the presence of a global auditory or visual 'weakness' having clear implications for speculations about the reading system which a child had established. The causal link between 'visual memory', 'auditory memory' or other aspects of intelligence and reading functions is too tenuous and too poorly validated to make this kind of indirect diagnosis seem anything other than an inadequate substitute for a direct cognitive analysis.

Rather similar comments appear applicable to discussions of dyslexia which are based on physiological indicators (Level III descriptions). Aside from indices of brain function, like the EEG, these consist of the results of psychophysical tests of sensory functions, e.g. audiometric assessments, tests of visual adequacy, including the establishment of a stable reference eye, eye-movement recordings, and other information, such as dominance of motor functions, handedness, incidence of learning disabilities within the family, or perinatal and subsequent medical history. It is desirable, in the interests of the compilation of comprehensive case descriptions, that information of this type should be tabulated. However, there is at present no principled or adequately validated basis for the assumption that the presence of a given Level III indicator implies any particular functional organisation of the reading process.

These remarks are intended to suggest that studies of dyslexia which are carried out using Level I indicators alone, or Level I indicators in conjunction with Level III indicators, have a limited value in the context of attempts to establish a diagnostically useful account of disordered reading functions. Indicators at these levels cannot confidently be used as substitutes for a properly detailed Level II (cognitive) analysis. It did not seem profitable to labour this point when discussing the data of the individual cases. However, I think it is clear that the Level II descriptions stand as direct analyses of currently available reading functions which are independent of and not directly predictable from the Level I and Level III information contained in the reports.

9.3   Treatment of data

The objective of establishing a procedure for the cognitive description of dyslexia raised a number of issues of methodology. The first of these concerned the problem of defining an appropriate level at which the data derived from experimental tests on subjects should be analysed. There seemed to be three possible approaches: (1) a standard experimental procedure in which subjects are assembled in groups and the data are analysed on a group basis; (2) a neuropsychological method, involving the identification of interesting cases and the analysis of individual data; and (3) a compromise approach requiring the investigation of similarities and differences existing among the individually analysed members of a subject sample.

The first approach was rejected on the grounds that it was based on an assumption in favour of the homogeneity of reading functions within samples of competent and disabled readers. The data, by showing wide ranging individual differences in performance indicators and processing configurations, suggest that the homogeneity assumption cannot be upheld and thus support the rejection of its associated methodology.

The second approach was also rejected. It seemed that a policy of restricting study to interesting or special cases introduced an unwanted bias into the process of subject selection. Further, the practice of treating individual case studies as prototype descriptions of dyslexic sub-types appeared hazardous in the absence of supportive data.

The research method which derived from these considerations involved: (1) the assembly of a subject sample, possibly linked to a particular organisation or institution, without the imposition of selective criteria; (2) the application of a common experimental procedure to all members of the sample; (3) the analysis of the results of each subject on an individual basis. These individual analyses resulted in the formulation of a series of interpretations (cognitive descriptions) which were expressed in the terminology of the information processing model which had been adopted as a framework for the research.

The cognitive descriptions provide a functional analysis of the reading of each member of the sample which is of potential value in diagnostic and remedial applications. The process of drawing more general conclusions, such as the adjudication between the sub-type and heterogeneity models of the distribution of dyslexic disorders, involves comparisons between descriptions of members of the sample, and the identification of similarities and differences.

9.4   **Experimental procedure**

An important aspect of the research method was the proposal that reading functions might best be studied by an adaptation of procedures which had been developed in mainstream cognitive experimental psychology. This method was defined as one in which linguistic stimuli are selected by sampling from categorised natural language subsets and are presented for naming or decision under specific task instructions and display conditions so as to allow for the accurate measurement of reaction time and the recording of response accuracy and other characteristics. This method is standard in cognitive psychology, but has in the past typically been applied to subject groups rather than to individuals.

I suggested that the time and accuracy data could be used in two ways. The evaluative usage involves a contrast between a subject's results and guidelines defining limits of efficient performance. Provided that the reference of the data to the model is clear, this usage allows the status of particular systems or pathways to be assessed as efficient or, to varying degrees, impaired. The second usage was interpretative and depended on the possibility of inferring characteristics of an individual's processing systems or overall configuration from a study of the effects of factor variations having a presumed localised reference in the model.

Part of the argument of this monograph has been that this type of experimental analysis is potentially informative in the diagnosis of dyslexic problems and might be preferred to other procedures, for example those which rely solely on accuracy scores or on conclusions which can be drawn from a classification of error types. In the present study much of the information about system status and function came from a consideration of the shapes of reaction time distributions and the occurrence of effects of the processing and psycholinguistic factors on reaction time levels.

9.5   **Competent reading**

In Chapter 5 I presented the results of a study of the reading functions of a small sample of competent 11-year-old readers. It is clearly desirable that this type of investigation should be carried out on a large scale and that a table of norms for the information processing tasks should be established for children of varying age, intelligence and reading competence. However, the sample turned out to contain quite considerable variability of reading function and thus probably gives a reasonable indication of the kinds of results which might be obtained from a larger group.

One difficulty in treating the data of the competent readers was posed by the discovery that formal competence is not incompatible with the occurrence of minor localised inefficiencies. Two approaches to the identification of these effects were adopted. One was based on the idea that the shapes of the reaction time distributions obtained in the different tasks could be treated as absolute indicators of efficiency, with a Type B distribution being taken as a sign of a mild inefficiency and a Type C distribution as a mark of a severe inefficiency. The second was the proposal that the error or reaction time levels which appeared to lie well outside the main set of scores presented by the competent reader sample should be treated as being indicative of a possible inefficiency.

If this standpoint is adopted, the results can be taken as evidence against the proposal that normal readers form a homogeneous group. This homogeneity presumption is opposed by the observation that some members of the sample exhibited localised inefficiencies in (1) accuracy of non-word reading, (2) latency of non-word reading, (3) latency of word reading, or (4) speed of analytic visual matching.

The analyses of the effects of the processing and psycholinguistic factors additionally suggested the existence of strategic variations between subjects. This conclusion depended on the possibility of treating the presence or absence of statistically significant effects as demonstrations of the occurrence or non-occurrence of the process associated with the factor in question. It was acknowledged that the inclusion of outlying reaction times in the analyses could work against the discovery of significant effects and the practice of removing times from the tails of Type B distributions was accordingly adopted.

The results suggested that the competent readers differed from one another strategically in a number of respects, including (1) the involvement of grapheme-phoneme and semantic processing in word retrieval, (2) the lexicalisation of output from the grapheme-phoneme channel, (3) the adoption of a serial self-terminating procedure in matching, (4) use of a serial procedure in format distortion resolution, and (5) speed-accuracy trading in making lexical decisions.

These results favour the conclusion that the information processing underlying competent reading is heterogeneous in distribution. An implication is that groups of competent readers who are employed as controls in studies of reading disability should be analysed on the same individual basis as has been proposed for samples of dyslexic cases.

9.6   Distribution of dyslexic impairments

The analysis of the result from the members of the dyslexic series was also indicative of large differences in the distribution and extent of inefficiencies and in the choice of processing options. A first conclusion, therefore, is that developmental dyslexia is not a homogeneous category. This excludes a model which assumes the existence of a single adverse factor which produces a consistent set of impairments within the processing system. It also serves as a justification for the individual case methodology which has been advocated and followed in this research.

The next question to consider is whether the cognitive descriptions of the dyslexic cases can usefully be grouped into a manageable number of distinctively defined sub-types. I have taken the notion of a sub-type to be applicable to the overall processing configuration presented by a subject. The configuration refers to the distribution of impairments across the systems postulated in the model and to the strategic options which have been adopted. A sub-type analysis might be favoured if it could be shown (1) that certain impairments occurred in a 'pure' form, or (2) that a dominant impairment tended to be accompanied by a specific pattern of lesser impairments and strategic compensations.

A classification based on the identities of 'pure' impairments has limited value since isolated dyslexias occurred only rarely and in subjects whose reading competence was high. Examples are the effects on route 'g' shown by AD and SS and by subjects JK and JS from the competent reader sample, and the visual processor effects shown by RO and the normal reader LH.

The data suggest, therefore, that cognitive analyses of dyslexic cases will most frequently yield evidence of multiple impairments. These could be viewed as independent effects or as correlated effects. According to the independence model each domain of the processing system might appear efficient or impaired to a variable degree, allowing for the occurrence of a large number of particular configurations. If the impairments were correlated, a major effect in one domain would tend to be accompanied by a particular pattern of effects in the other domains.

In the discussion of the cases, an attempt was made to explore the applicability of a model assuming correlation of effects. According to one version of this model, an adverse influence in one domain will have a large disruptive effect on that process combined with a scatter of consequent effects and strategic adjustments in the other domains. There were some associations in the data which appeared arguably consistent with such a theory. For example, both visual processor and morphemic impairments were generally accompanied by some effects on route 'g'. However, it is in practice difficult to distinguish these concurrences from all the other associations which occurred in the data of some subjects but not of others. No firm conclusion can be based on the absence of a dissociation in one sample of subjects since the dissociation may well turn up in the next sample which is studied.

For these reasons, I do not consider that the data can easily be fitted into a coherent scheme of sub-types. To do this it would be desirable to be able to identify categories of 'visual processor dyslexia', 'phonological dyslexia' and 'morphemic dyslexia' and to define these by reference to their primary impairment and the associated effects and strategies. If this is attempted with the present sample, a majority of subjects are found to belong to more than one category and the pattern of accompanying effects appears markedly inconsistent.

It is probably wisest, therefore, to retain a model which allows for the independent impairment of each domain. According to this theory, the domains may be degraded separately or in combination. The cognitive description which is derived will depend on how widespread and how severe the domain-specific degradation is. Thus, the status of a particular domain must be assumed to reflect intrinsic properties of its neural substrate rather than variations in the quality of the information which it receives from other parts of the processing system.

A methodological implication is that a cognitive assessment should always involve an experimental analysis of each of the major domains of the model. The demonstration that a particular process is impaired cannot be assumed to carry reliable implications about the status of the other systems and processes.

As was noted earlier, the independence model has implications for the usage of the term 'dyslexia' in a cognitive analysis. The term has to be treated as descriptive of impaired processes or domains and not of processing configurations. Thus, the expression 'phonological dyslexia' might mean that route 'g' was impaired although it would not be taken to imply anything about the states of the other systems.

9.7 Visual processor dyslexia

Some of the subjects gave evidence of an inefficiency localised within the visual processor. I have referred to this effect as 'visual processor dyslexia'. However, it would be incorrect to regard this category as equivalent to formally similar designations deriving from other diagnostic schemes, such as 'visual dyslexia' or 'dyseidetic dyslexia'. Indeed, if it is correct to regard the visual processor as a graphemic specialist which is functionally distinct from other visual analysers, it follows that tests involving object perception or visual memory for non-linguistic materials may have little bearing on the status of the visual processor required for reading.

Stein and Fowler (1982) have argued that the absence of a stable reference eye may be a critical factor in producing a visual form of dyslexia. This matter was not systematically investigated in the present study. However, the data do not encourage the view that 'visual processor dyslexia', as defined here, will typically be accompanied by evidence of an unstable reference eye. Subjects who showed large visual processor effects, such as MF, CE, SE and PS, had fixed reference eyes. Other subjects who were classified as unfixed, including LA and JB, did not give evidence of visual processor inefficiency.

In the model the visual processor was defined as a complex system which incorporated a number of levels, including (1) a level of letter identification, and (2) a level of parsing and data transfer. The first level was assessed by means of the identity matching task and the second by the array matching task and by the variations in word length and format which were built into the experiments. It was additionally proposed that the processor internalises a model of English orthographic structure which can be used to facilitate array matching and negative responses in lexical decision experiments.

A general assumption, deriving from Shallice's (1981) distinction between 'attentional dyslexia' and 'word-form dyslexia', was that the processor might transfer data in a wholistic or in an analytic/segmental mode. What has here been called 'visual processor dyslexia' or 'visual analytic dyslexia' was seen as an inefficiency affecting the analytic mode of the processor. The characteristic features appeared to be: (1) very slow reaction times when making 'same'-'different' judgments about pairs of letter arrays, and (2) very slow serial processing when reading vertically distorted words (cf. RO, MF, CE, MT and PS). For some subjects the effect extended to the reaction time in the identity matching task, but this was not invariably the case.

The effect can be interpreted as a processing delay which will be evident whenever the visual processor is forced to operate in an analytic mode. This mode may be obligatory for point-by-point comparison between arrays, detection of identity under conditions of poor discriminability, the spatial recoding of distorted displays, and the graphemic segmentation of arrays prior to phonological recoding via route 'g'. Where analytic processing is not required, as in the reading of normally formatted familiar words, reading may appear quite efficient, provided that no higher order dyslexias are present.

This analysis depends on some assumptions about the manner in which distorted formats are resolved. These include the proposals (1) that the recognition level of the processor is adapted to the identification of arrays incorporating a horizontal spatial coding oriented from left to right, and (2) that information is represented at the identity level of the processor in a spatial code which defines the actual distribution of elements on the display. Format resolution is seen as a process of spatial reorganisation by which codes representing vertical location and direction are replaced by equivalent horizontal descriptors. It is assumed that this is carried out at the parsing level of the processor and that it requires an analytic mode in which letter identities are selected one at a time for redescription.

Subjects showing evidence of a visual analytic dyslexia tended also to exhibit slow serial reading of non-words. This was taken to suggest that an effect on the analytic mode of the processor will usually have some adverse consequences for the operation of route 'g'. This constitutes an exception to the independence assumption, since it involves the proposal that an analytic impairment implies an associated impairment in the grapheme-phoneme route to phonology. In the case of RO, non-words were accurately read and the distribution was well formed although the processing rate was in excess of 200 ms/letter. This suggests a limitation on the speed of analytic functioning in the absence of a higher order phonological dyslexia. The other subjects all showed more substantial phonological effects in which serial processing was combined with general evidence of inefficiency in route 'g'. Given that RO's visual processor disturbance was so large, it is probably wisest to interpret the phonological effects shown by MF, CE, MT and PS as joint products of the analytic disturbance and an independence impairment of the phonological processor. Nonetheless, it would not be surprising if the earlier development of route 'g' was limited by the presence of a visual analytic disturbance. This relationship could be assessed by studies of younger dyslexic subjects.

A further possibility is that the analytic impairment may affect the acquisition of spelling knowledge. This issue lies outside the scope of the present work since its investigation requires a careful within-subject comparison between reading patterns and spelling patterns. However, it is clear that a defect of analytic processing could be incompatible with careful attention to the detail of spelling structure. This might lead to an inadequately lexicalised spelling system characterised by the production of phonetically accurate mis-spellings. In the cases of RO and MF the analytic impairment did not prevent the internalisation of orthographic knowledge within the visual processor, since both subjects showed effects of legality in the matching and lexical decision tasks.

9.8 Morphemic dyslexia

A 'morphemic dyslexia' has been defined as an impairment affecting one or both of the 'm' routes to phonology or semantics. The effect is marked by high error rates and slow responses (Type B or C distributions) in word reading tasks. Issues which have arisen in the earlier discussions are: (1) whether or not the two 'm' routes can be independently impaired; (2) whether morphemic dyslexia derives from a disturbance of the wholistic function of the visual processor; (3) whether the impairment forces the adoption of a compensatory strategy involving reliance on reading via route 'g'; and (4) whether a morphemic impairment implies an accompanying effect on the efficiency of grapheme-phoneme translation.

An effect on route 'm' to semantics could arise because the semantic processor was itself degraded or because of some inefficiency in the process of accessing or retrieving semantic information. An impoverished semantic processor should be marked by low scores on the verbal scales of the Wechsler intelligence tests, and by inaccurate performance on the semantic categorisation task, especially for items of low typicality (cf. subject LH). A limitation due to impaired access processes seems more likely to be marked by an elevation of the reaction time levels for semantic decisions (cf. subjects LA, SM and GS).

The information provided by the lexical decision task is more difficult to interpret. One problem is that some of the competent readers were willing to tolerate high error rates, especially on the legal non-words. This means that a high false positive rate on these items cannot be treated as an indication of a morphemic effect. Further, if a subject adopts a strategy of responding positively to orthographically legal arrays, the acceptance rates for words will appear spuriously high. Consequently, the lexical decision results are worth treating as an index of a morphemic effect only if incorrect responses to words occur in the context of reasonably accurate performance on legal non-words. It might then be arguable that a high false rejection rate implied that only a restricted range of vocabulary was represented in the morphemic recognition space of the visual processor.

More fundamental problems are posed by the existence of theoretical uncertainties about the manner in which lexical decisions are made. One possibility is that the decision is taken at the level of the morpheme recognition space in the visual processor. A second is that positive decisions depend on the retrieval of semantic (or phonological) information. Depending on which view is correct, reaction time delays in classification of words will reflect slowness in accessing the recognition space or slowness in retrieving higher order information.

The morphemic route to phonology was assessed in the tasks involving the vocalisation of high and low frequency words. An effect on accuracy could occur (1) because the range of vocabulary stored within the phonological processor was limited, or (2) because there were restrictions on the scope of the morpheme recognition space. An effect on vocal reaction time is suggestive of problems in accumulating information for recognition or in accessing and retrieving lexical phonological codes.

The results suggested that the two routes were potentially dissociable. Although the effects often extended to both routes, some subjects (e.g. LT) demonstrated an impairment of route 'm' to phonology in the absence of a corresponding effect on route 'm' to semantics. The opposed dissociation, an effect on the semantic route in the absence of an effect on the phonological route, did not occur in this sample. However, the subject BS, tested by Seymour and Porpodas (1980), may be a case in point. This subject read non-words extremely slowly (mean RT over 11,000 ms) but read words accurately with a latency below 800 ms, suggesting the absence of an effect on route 'm' to phonology. He did not undertake a semantic categorisation experiment. However, his performance in a lexical decision task was extremely impaired, with the RT well in excess of 4000 ms, and an error rate rising to over 20 per cent on lower frequency words despite accurate responses to legal non-words.

A practical implication of these results is that it will always be advisable to assess morphemic dyslexia by making tests on the status of both the semantic and the phonological routes. Theoretically, the dissociation raises questions about the level at which the two processes become differentiated from one another. One possibility, argued by Seymour and MacGregor (1984), is that there are two distinct lexical recognition spaces, one giving access to semantics and the other to phonology. However, this idea was based on the suggestion that access to semantics relied on a primitive whole word recognition system (the logographic lexicon) whereas access to phonology involved a sophisticated version of the grapheme-phoneme channel (referred to as the 'orthographic lexicon'). Such an account is consistent with the results of subjects like LT and SB, who exhibited efficient functioning in the semantic route combined with a major effect on route 'g' and a relatively milder effect on route 'm' to phonology. However, it is difficult to square with the results of Seymour and Porpodas's subject BS, since the theory assumes that efficiency in route 'g' is a necessary prerequisite for the construction of an orthographic lexicon.

On these grounds, it may be desirable to retain the proposal that the visual processor contains a single morpheme recognition space which mediates access to the phonological processor or to the semantic processor. According to this theory, morphemic effects which differed in magnitude could be localised in the routes themselves or at the level of access to the higher level processors.

A related set of issues is raised by the suggestion that morphemic dyslexia may be a consequence of an impairment of the wholistic function of the visual processor. The general hypothesis here is that a disordered wholistic process results in a reliance on an analytic processing mode which is inimical to the development of a morpheme recognition system while being favourable to the establishment of a grapheme-phoneme translation channel. If this theory was correct it would be expected that morphemic dyslexia should be associated with evidence of slow serial processing in all reading tasks. Some subjects, most particularly SM, showed a pattern of this kind. However, there were many exceptions and it was often the case that serial processing was more strongly apparent for the phonological tasks than for the lexical and semantic tasks. If serial processing is dependent on the higher order route which is being accessed, it becomes unlikely that it can be viewed as an intrinsic property of the visual processor and more probable that it is a response to demands of the higher level access channel.

There seem to be two ways in which the higher functions could dictate whether or not the parsing process operated in a serial mode. One idea might be to return to the dual lexicon proposal, as put forward by Seymour and MacGregor (1984), and to argue that access to phonology via the orthographic lexicon generally requires some analytic or segmental processing whereas access to semantics via a logographic lexicon can be achieved by wholistic processing. The alternative is to stand by the arguments in favour of a single morpheme recognition space and to accept that serial processing may, optionally, be involved during access. A likely possibility is that serial processing is a property of route 'g' and will be evident whenever grapheme-phoneme translation is used as a back-up for the morpheme recognition process.

This leads on to the question of whether morphemic dyslexia can confidently be associated with a compensatory strategy which involves a reliance on processing via route 'g'. Since the adoption of such a strategy will be marked by (1) the occurrence of effects of spelling-to-sound regularity, and (2) the production of non-word error responses which include phonetic regularisations, this is mainly a question about the signs which might be used to identify a morphemic dyslexic sub-type. The present results suggest that this kind of analysis cannot be made without considering the status of the 'g' route to phonology. A frequently recurring configuration is one in which a morphemic dyslexia is combined with an impairment of route 'g' although the balance of severity of the two effects may vary. There were some subjects, most notably SM, GS and LH, who appeared to read in this way, and others, such as LT and JB, who did not. It seems likely that these are the extremes of a continuum which is determined by the balance of impairment in routes 'g' and 'm' and perhaps by strategic choices which may be influenced by instruction. For this reason it seems preferable to treat the regularity effects as an index of strategy rather than as a mark of the presence of a morphemic dyslexia which can more appropriately be defined by direct tests on the efficiency of the 'm' routes.

In this sample it was invariably the case that morphemic impairments were accompanied by evidence of inefficiency in route 'g'. If this finding is sustained in other samples and no valid exceptions are forthcoming, the implication will be that the development of route 'g' is contingent on the establishment of an adequate lexical base. However, wider sampling seems necessary before this potentially significant modification to the independence model might be thought to merit general acceptance.

9.9 Phonological dyslexia

All of the subjects in the dyslexic sample gave some evidence of 'phonological dyslexia', defined in terms of inaccuracy or reaction time delays in reading non-words. Phonological effects also occurred in the sample of competent readers. The effect varied greatly in severity and affected accuracy, reaction time or both.

The accuracy effect will be considered first. Probably the most important point is that all of the subjects in the sample possessed operational grapheme-phoneme translation channels and were able to read non-words with reasonable success. Correct readings occurred for 60 per cent of items or more, and errors were usually fairly close approximations to the target involving inaccurate translation of vowels or minor faults of letter identification or order. In most instances responses were based on simple grapheme-phoneme correspondences.

The striking feature of the route 'g' impairment was the occurrence of substantial reaction time delays in the production of responses to non-words. These effects were often related to non-word length and involved large increases in reaction time for each additional letter which was translated. In some cases, processing was further slowed by the presence of format distortions. Some subjects were able to reduce their reaction time or improve accuracy when responding to non-words which were homophones of English words.

The construction of a grapheme-phoneme translation channel probably depends on a capacity to segment speech into phonemic units and to identify the graphemic clusters to which they reliably correspond. Since the subjects all demonstrated the availability of a moderately effective channel, it is arguable that these prerequisites were satisfied. The errors and slow reactions might then reflect imprecision in the mapping from grapheme to phoneme or a delay in carrying out an operation of phonological retrieval rather than a lack of a fundamental 'phonemic awareness'.

It is possible that Level I indicators such as the digit span or the Lindamood Auditory Conceptualisation test tap difficulties localised within the phonological processor which can give rise to impairments of the grapheme-phoneme channel. However, it is evident from the case studies that the relationship between these tests and the degree of impairment of route 'g' is somewhat variable. For example, subjects GS and MP had very low scores on the Lindamood test but were fairly accurate in reading non-words. It seems that it is preferable to assess the status of route 'g' directly by applying a non-word reading task in which reaction times are measured rather than by relying on tests which may engage other resources of the processor.

The results are not sufficiently analytic to support a detailed account of the disturbance of route 'g' in individual cases. Part of the problem is that it is difficult to partial out the contributions of the different possible stages in grapheme-phoneme translation. A visual contribution could arise if the processor had failed to internalise vowel and consonant orthographic structures or if there were limitations on its rate of parsing letter arrays into small graphemic clusters. Arguments to suggest that these aspects were not generally important can be derived from the observations: (1) most subjects gave evidence of internalisation of orthographic structure, either in matching or in lexical decisions or in both; (2) the processing rates observed in non-word reading were often substantially slower than those observed in word reading; and (3) difficulty with complex clusters was often greater for vowels than for consonants. At the same time, it was often true that the slow processing rates observed in non-word reading were exaggerated by the presence of format distortions. One way of interpreting these observations is to suggest that the route 'g' impairment was not directly consequent on any defect in the visual processor, but that the rate at which the processor could operate was limited by the slowness of the higher level retrieval and assembly functions, and this effect was liable to interact with any additional load imposed by the distortions.

The central stage of grapheme-phoneme conversion can plausibly be represented as involving (1) the retrieval of phonemic elements, and (2) the assembly of the elements into an appropriately ordered sequence. Defects in either or both of these processes could give rise to inaccuracies and delays in non-word reading. Thus, 'phonological dyslexia' could be represented as an inefficiency affecting the retrieval and/or assembly of phonemic elements. The special difficulty with complex vowels is most obviously interpreted as an effect on retrieval. It is not easy to estimate the contribution of the response organisation phase. However, one possibility is that the homophony effect operates on this stage. This would occur if the transmission of discrete phonemes to the vocabulary store resulted in the retrieval of an integrated response, thus bypassing the need for ordering and assembly operations. Nonetheless, it is probably right to view the homophony effect as an index of strategy (a readiness to refer phonemic elements to the speech production lexicon) rather than as a measure of difficulty in the assembly stage of translation.

The relationship between the grapheme-phoneme channel and the morphemic channels remains obscure. According to the independence model, the channel is a distinct system which may be developmentally impaired if its neural substrate is degraded. This impairment is not considered to be a consequence of an impairment in another system. Nor is it supposed to carry consequences for the development of other systems. Nonetheless, there was a preponderance of cases in whom impairments of the 'm' and 'g' routes were combined. It is at present difficult to choose between an account in which 'neural degradation' typically extends across routes and one in which a measure of functional interdependence is assumed.

9.10   Implications for diagnosis and remediation

The cognitive assessment procedure offers a more precise and sensitive method of describing the reading processes of dyslexic subjects than the traditional techniques currently available to teachers and educational psychologists. The procedure is at present in the form of a research tool and would need development before it could become established as a diagnostic instrument. Some limitations are:

(1)   the procedure is designed for investigation of dyslexia in older subjects and would require modification before it could be used with younger children;

(2)   the procedure is adapted for the study of individuals who have achieved a partial competence in reading and would be of limited use with children who were effectively non-readers;

(3)   a more extensive 'normative base' is required.

However, these are primarily matters of a practical nature which could be dealt with by widening and differentiating the application of the method. I see no reason in principle why cognitive theories should not be combined with microcomputer technology to produce a useful diagnostic technique which could beneficially be introduced to supplement existing procedures.

The cognitive method carried with it a set of assumptions about reading processes which were set out at the beginning of this monograph. The key ideas were (1) that reading can be represented in terms of a functionally defined modular system, and (2) that information about processing modules can be gained by applications of the experimental method. It will have been evident from the case studies that these assumptions play a critical role in determining the diagnostic categories which can be proposed. Diagnosis has to be expressed in the form of references to hypothetical processing systems and routes, and these references depend on certain conventions of interpretation which relate experimental observations to the workings of the model.

In the present study, diagnosis was seen as a matter of attempting to set up probing techniques which could be used to examine the status of the systems and routes postulated in the model. This led to the formulation of 'cognitive descriptions' of each subject's reading processes. These descriptions may be treated individually as diagnostic statements about the distribution of impairments within a single subject.

A question of importance was whether diagnosis should be carried forward to a superordinate level of analysis at which cognitive descriptions could be compared, contrasted and grouped into categories. This approach would be justified if the descriptions obtained from the members of the subject sample fell into a small number of clearly defined and theoretically intelligible subsets, each of which could then be proposed as a 'dyslexic sub-type'. The idea of a sub-type was seen to be based on the recurrence of a particular distribution of impairments and strategic compensations.

The viability of a sub-type analysis is likely to be dependent on the size and origins of the subject sample providing the cognitive descriptions. The conclusion from the present study was that the descriptions of the 21 subjects were somewhat heterogeneous, and that the applicability of a sub-type analysis had not been demonstrated.

This conclusion has theoretical and practical implications. It has been used to support a model of dyslexia in which it is assumed that component processing systems and routes may be independently impaired. The idea of independence carries with it the suggestion that the causal basis of the impairment may be intrinsic to the neural substrate of the affected system. At a practical level, it is suggested that diagnosis should involve an attempt to assess the status of each of a number of processing components, and not an assignment of a subject to a sub-type category.

The longer-term objective of a theoretical and diagnostic analysis of dyslexia is the improvement of the possibilities of remediation. Most of the subjects in the present sample had received substantial amounts of help, both through their schools and through private tuition, and had, in many cases, achieved educational success and gone a long way towards overcoming their reading difficulties. Unfortunately, the properties of this remedial input are not sufficiently well defined to permit any statements about the teaching techniques which proved effective in particular cases.

The evaluation of remedial techniques is a topic for future research. What is required is a clear definition of the teaching method together with some explicit assumptions about the component of the information processing system which is likely to be affected, and the nature of the expected effect. It might then be possible to use the cognitive assessment procedure to determine whether or not a method was successful in improving the status of a particular system or route.

If remediation is to take account of the diagnostic information provided by a cognitive assessment, it seems desirable that some techniques having a selective and localised reference should be established. Using the analysis of the four domains, these would include (1) a method of improving the operational efficiency of the visual processor, (2) a method of influencing accuracy or speed of translation via route 'g', and (3) procedures for expanding the scope of the morpheme recognition system and of improving the speed or precision of access to phonology and semantics via the 'm' routes.

From the standpoint of the competence analysis of reading, the most critical issue concerns the status of the morphemic components. The public definition of 'dyslexia' is stated in terms of an individual's lack of competence in pronouncing and comprehending meaningful written language. Hence, 'dyslexia' will generally involve an impairment of the 'm' routes, and its remediation will require the application of procedures which are capable of influencing the morphemic processes. It is not at present clear exactly what these procedures might be, but it seems likely that the routes to phonology and semantics may need independent treatment and that a method of highlighting morphemic structure might be helpful.

Traditionally, dyslexia has been treated by regimes which emphasise a structured approach to phonic analysis. It is very possible that these procedures have a number of side effects, such as improvement of spelling knowledge, development of morpheme recognition and internalisation of orthographic information in the visual processor. However, if the technique functions solely as an influence on route 'g', its contribution to the solution of morphemic difficulties may be quite limited. What may be achieved is an encouragement to use the translation process as a support for word retrieval via the morphemic route. The results made it clear that back-up processing of this kind was widely resorted to, even by subjects giving evidence of quite severe route 'g' impairments. An implication is, perhaps, that phonics-oriented remediation could usefully emphasise the possibilities of a two-way interaction between the 'm' and 'g' routes.

9.11   Summary and conclusions

The purpose of this monograph has been to explain and illustrate a particular approach to the analysis of the reading disorders which may be encountered in cases of developmental dyslexia. The main argument has been that there is merit in attempting to analyse dyslexia at a level of underlying cognitive processes, and that the achievement of this goal requires:

(1)   the specification of a functional model of basic reading processes;
(2)   the design of an experimental procedure capable of probing the status of the components of the model; and
(3)   the application of the procedure to the individual members of samples of competent and dyslexic readers.

The empirical section of the monograph consisted of competence descriptions, experimental data and cognitive descriptions of the members of a small group of normal readers and of 21 subjects having histories of dyslexic problems. It was proposed that reading functions could be described by reference to four domains represented in the functional model: (1) a visual processor specialised for the analysis of print; (1) a morphemic route to semantics; (3) a morphemic route to phonology; and (4) a grapheme-phoneme translation route to phonology.

The results suggested that the members of both samples exhibited variations in the efficiency and the strategic organisation of the processing domains. It was concluded that developmental dyslexia was not a homogeneous category and that the cases were not amenable to classification into a small number of clearly defined sub-types. A model allowing for the independent impairment of the different processing domains appeared to be tenable. A diagnostic approach involving the separate assessment and remediation of each domain was advised.

Appendix 1 Word lists

(1) *List varying form class and abstract concrete meaning*

High frequency words

Concrete
car boy pen fur bar gun egg paper stone cabin wheat tower hotel clock
village machine diamond railway chicken curtain picture

Abstract
age aim act sin fun wit aid anger charm faith shame sleep power delay
history society benefit respect variety average liberty

Function words
the her all any and but for per why him how not off too these where after
which about those since every among until whose below above again
because himself without through between against several whether someone
herself anybody however already another

Low frequency words

Concrete
dam ale pod gem cud ram keg toast puppy acorn spray poker tonic whale
volcano lantern admiral leaflet reptile sunburn spinach

Abstract
fad par rot era kin fee gap agony drama green panic dogma irony spree
anger charm economy loyalty heroism phantom concept disgust agility

(2) *List varying spelling-to-sound regularity*

High frequency words

Regular
art end oil out pay tea win army bone hand life soon term wing brown

brush cheap house limit mount order compel forget happen insist little pocket winter

Irregular
any eye key one two who won come debt love aunt shoe sign blow blood money water laugh ought prove touch answer beauty cousin island listen people tongue

Low frequency words

Regular
elm gap mar mug sly bud yon chin dive hike hawk peel epic wink acute brood canon snore drunk grill quest groove export juggle modest porter pistol racket

Irregular
aye guy mow gem ski tow yea ache bomb comb heir boy hymn wasp aisle bough dwarf corps chasm quart rhyme eighth quartz legion orchid martyr plough resign

Appendix 2   Non-word lists

(1)   *List varying non-word homophony*

Homophones

lor slo wor woz hiz oke kar jin ise lim yoo doo joi owt hoo kee boi boe toi
hai wurry sivic ampul lojic wurld klock dijit jipsy tabel ajent pawse furst
sleap shaim brawd pownd creem scrue eezel howse konsent biznes sentury
phashun sentrul citizun jymnast orchurd lettiss actruss fealing cawshun
kleerly brorden becawse masheen awction teecher pengwin ranebow

Non-homophones

lar plo vor foz hoz uke dar jun ose bim fod doi jow owb noo ree goi voe
taw vai nurry givic umpul lijic murld kleck sijit jepsy habel ejent dawse surst
slaip sheam broid cownd freem scrow oozel bowse kansent lizness sintury
phoshun bentrul litizun pymnast archurd dettis octruss jealing ceashun
klairly trorden secawse mashoon aiction toicher tengwin fanebow

(2)   *List varying lexical environment*

Consistent regular environment

blax lelt otch grox nusk inge screp crift sitch ackle spumb fedge spleck trinch
bupple thrunt quodge mamble clak relp idge smup noft adge streb frisp
sonch uggle snelk pupon thralp trunge fletal squilk privel voddle

Consistently irregular environment

galk vold aven enal inal ocal dach ipen onge utal apon iten ation fralm
prolk dason nidal gotal yaden tiden popen gucal foval mital kotion sprild
strolt twegal sniral chodal plaval breden twival flonal whugal spluth

Inconsistent environment with a regular bias

clon nint vull scrut blonk phush flutch squant stross whas drix molf throm
scuss bavel wabble friven thovel

Inconsistent environment with an irregular bias

palt gind ange prall thost soven throll scroth storal rald balf ison frimb shomb meven rasten shront slanal

Influence of initial /w/

twap wamp squan whash quatch squath

(from Maccabe, 1984)

References

Beauvois, M.F. and Derouesne, J. (1979), 'Phonological alexia: three dissociations', *Journal of Neurology, Neurosurgery and Psychiatry*, *42*, pp. 115-25.

Beller, H.K. (1970), 'Parallel and serial stages in matching', *Journal of Experimental Psychology*, *84*, pp. 213-19.

Boder, E. (1973, 'Developmental dyslexia: a diagnostic approach based on three atypical reading-spelling patterns', *Developmental Medicine and Child Neurology*, *21*, pp. 504-14.

Bryant, P.E. and Bradley, L. (1980), 'Why children sometimes write words which they do not read', in Frith, U. (ed.), *Cognitive Processes in Spelling*, London, Academic Press.

Chambers, S.M. and Forster, K.I. (1975), 'Evidence for lexical access in a simultaneous matching task', *Memory and Cognition*, *3*, pp. 549-59.

Coltheart, M. (1978), 'Lexical access in simple reading tasks', in Underwood, G. (ed.), *Strategies of Information Processing*, London, Academic Press.

Coltheart, M. (1980), 'Deep dyslexia: a review of the syndrome,' in Coltheart, M., Patterson, K. and Marshall, J.C. (eds), *Deep Dyslexia*, London, Routledge & Kegan Paul.

Coltheart, M., Masterson, J., Byng, S., Prior, M. and Riddoch, J. (1983), 'Surface dyslexia', *Quarterly Journal of Experimental Psychology*, *35A*, pp. 469-95.

Critchley, M. (1970), *The Dyslexic Child*, London, Heinemann.

Frith, U. (1985), 'Beneath the surface of developmental dyslexia', in Patterson, K.E., Marshall, J.C. and Coltheart, M. (eds), *Surface Dyslexia: Neuropsychological and Cognitive Analyses of Phonological Reading*, London, Lawrence Erlbaum Associates.

Geschwind, N. (1965), 'Disconnexion syndromes in animals and man', *Brain*, *88*, pp. 237-94.

Gibson, E.J., Pick, A., Osser, H. and Hammond, M. (1962), 'The role of grapheme-phoneme correspondence in the perception of words', *American*

Journal of Psychology, 75, pp. 554-70.

Glushko, R.J. (1979), 'The organisation and activation of orthographic knowledge in reading aloud', *Journal of Experimental Psychology: Human Perception and Performance*, 5, pp. 674-91.

Henderson, L. (1982), *Orthography and Word Recognition in Reading*, London, Academic Press.

Hinshelwood, J. (1917), *Congenital Word-blindness*, London, H.K. Lewis.

Johnson, D. and Myklebust, H. (1967), *Learning Disabilities: Educational Principles and Practices*, New York, Grune & Stratton.

Kucera, H. and Francis, W.N. (1967), *Computational Analysis of Present-day American English*, Providence, Rhode Island, Brown University Press.

Maccabe, I.D. (1984), 'Phonography: data and speculation', paper presented at a meeting of the Experimental Psychology Society, London.

Marsh, G., Friedman, M.P., Welch, V. and Desberg, P. (1981), 'A cognitive-developmental approach to reading acquisition', in Waller, T. and MacKinnon, G.E. (eds), *Reading Research: Advances in Theory and Practice, Volume 2*, New York, Academic Press.

Marshall, J.C. and Newcombe, F. (1973), 'Patterns of paralexia: a psycholinguistic approach', *Journal of Psycholinguistic Research*, 2, pp. 175-99.

Miles, T.R. (1983), *Dyslexia: The Pattern of Difficulties*, London, Granada.

Mitterer, J.O. (1982), 'There are at least two kinds of poor readers: whole word poor readers and recoding poor readers', *Canadian Journal of Psychology*, 36, pp. 445-61.

Morton, J. (1968), 'Grammar and computation in language behavior', Progress Report no. 6, Center for Research in Language and Language Behavior, University of Michigan, Ann Arbor, May 1968.

Morton, J. (1969), 'The interaction of information in word recognition', *Psychological Review*, 76, pp. 165-78.

Morton, J. and Patterson, K.E. (1980), 'A new attempt at an interpretation, or, an attempt at a new interpretation', in Coltheart, M., Patterson, K. and Marshall, J.C. (eds), *Deep Dyslexia*, London, Routledge & Kegan Paul.

Paivio, A., Yuille, J.C. and Madigan, S. (1968), 'Concreteness, imagery and meaningfulness values for 925 nouns', *Journal of Experimental Psychology Monograph*, 76 (1, Part 2).

Patterson, K.E. (1982), 'The relation between reading and phonological coding: further neuropsychological observations', in Ellis, A.W. (ed.), *Normality and Pathology in Cognitive Functioning*, London, Academic Press.

Patterson, K.E. and Morton, J. (1985), 'From orthography to phonology: an attempt at an old interpretation', in Patterson, K.E., Marshall, J.C. and Coltheart, M. (eds), *Surface Dyslexia: Neuropsychological and Cognitive Analyses of Phonological Reading*, London, Lawrence Erlbaum Associates.

Posner, M.I. and Mitchell, R.F. (1967), 'Chronometric analysis of classification', *Psychological Review*, *74*, pp. 392-409.

Rosch, E. (1975), 'Cognitive representation of semantic categories', *Journal of Experimental Psychology: General*, *104*, pp. 192-233.

Satz, P. and Morris, R. (1981), 'Learning disability sub-types: a review', in Pirozzolo, F.J. and Wittrock, M.C. (eds), *Neuropsychological and Cognitive Processes in Reading*, New York, Academic Press.

Seymour, P.H.K. (1973), 'A model for reading, naming and comparison', *British Journal of Psychology*, *64*, pp. 35-49.

Seymour, P.H.K. (1979), *Human Visual Cognition: A Study in Experimental Cognitive Psychology*, London: Collier Macmillan.

Seymour, P.H.K. (1985), 'Developmental dyslexia: a cognitive experimental analysis', in Coltheart, M., Job, R. and Sartori, G. (eds), *The Cognitive Neuropsychology of Language*, London, Lawrence Erlbaum Associates.

Seymour, P.H.K. and Elder, L. (1986), 'Beginning reading without phonology', *Cognitive Neuropsychology*, *3*, pp. 1-36.

Seymour, P.H.K. and MacGregor, C.J. (1984), 'Developmental dyslexia: a cognitive experimental analysis of phonological, morphemic and visual impairments', *Cognitive Neuropsychology*, *1*, pp. 43-82.

Seymour, P.H.K. and Porpodas, C.D. (1980), 'Lexical and non-lexical processing of spelling in dyslexia', in Frith, U. (ed.), *Cognitive Processes in Spelling*, London, Academic Press.

Shallice, T. (1981), 'Neurological impairment of cognitive processes', *British Medical Bulletin*, *27*, pp. 187-92.

Shallice, T. and Warrington, E.K. (1975), 'Word recognition in a phonemic dyslexic patient', *Quarterly Journal of Experimental Psychology*, *27*, pp. 187-199.

Shallice, T., Warrington, E.K. and McCarthy, R. (1983), 'Reading without semantics', *Quarterly Journal of Experimental Psychology*, *35A*, pp. 111-38.

Smith, E.E., Shoben, E.J. and Rips, L.J. (1974), 'Structure and process in semantic memory: a featural model for semantic decisions', *Psychological Review*, *81*, pp. 214-41.

Stein, J. and Fowler, S. (1982), 'Ocular motor dyslexia', *Dyslexia Review*, *5*, pp. 25-8.

Temple, C.M. and Marshall, J.C. (1983), 'A case study of developmental phonological dyslexia', *British Journal of Psychology*, *74*, pp. 517-33.

Thorndike, E.L. and Lorge, I. (1944), *The Teacher's Word Book of 30,000 Words*, New York, Columbia University Press.

Warren, C.E.J. and Morton, J. (1982), 'The effects of priming on picture recognition', *British Journal of Psychology*, *73*, pp. 117-30.

Sources for principal tests referred to in the psycho-educational assessments

Daniels, J.C. and Diack, H. (1973), *The Standard Reading Tests*, London: Chatto & Windus.

Graham, F.J. and Kendall, B.S. (1946), *Memory for Designs Test*, Windsor: NFER-Nelson.

Kirk, S.A. and McCarthy, J.J. (1968), *The Illinois Test of Psycholinguistic Abilities*, Urbana, Illinois: University of Illinois Press.

Lindamood, C.H. and Lindamood, PC. (1979), *Lindamood Auditory Conceptualisation Test*, Hingham, Mass.: Teaching Resources Corporation.

Miles, T.R. (1983), *Dyslexia: The Pattern of Difficulties*, London: Granada (Bangor Dyslexia Test).

Neale, M.D. (1966), *Neale Analysis of Reading Ability*, London: Macmillan.

Newton, M.J. and Thomson, M.E. (1976), *The Aston Index: A Screening Procedure for Written Language Difficulties*, Wisbech: Learning Development Aids.

Schonell, G.B. and Schonell, F.E. (1956), *Diagnostic and Attainment Testing*, Edinburgh: Oliver & Boyd.

Wechsler Adult Intelligence Scale (1957), New York: Psychological Corporation.

Wechsler Intelligence Scale for Children (Revised) (1976), Windsor: NFER-Nelson.

Wepman, J.M. (1975), *Auditory Discrimination Test*, Palm Springs, California: Language Research Associates.

Index

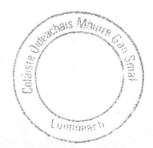